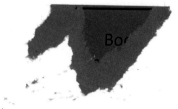

Bo

NHS FOR SALE

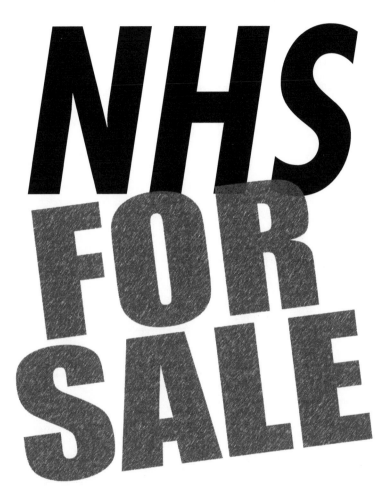

NHS FOR SALE

Myths, Lies & Deception

Jacky Davis, John Lister, David Wrigley

MERLIN PRESS

© Tamasin Cave, Jacky Davis, Paul Evans, John Lister,
Martin McKee, Harry Smith, David Wrigley, 2015

First published in 2015 by
The Merlin Press Ltd
99b Wallis Road
London
E9 5LN

www.merlinpress.co.uk

ISBN. 978-0-85036-627-3

British Library Cataloguing in Publication Data
is available from the British Library

Printed in the UK by Imprint Digital, Exeter

Contents

Acknowledgements

For much helpful and generous advice, our thanks go to Anna Athow, Prof. Colin Crouch, Prof. Colin Leys and Prof. Ray Tallis; we thank Peter Phillips and Glenda Pattenden for the cover concept and design, and tender particular thanks to Harry Smith for the foreword, Prof. Martin McKee for the introduction, and Tamasin Cave and Paul Evans for their contributions on the health lobbying industry and on NHS vital statistics under the coalition.

To the memory of Aneurin Bevan and to the frontline
NHS staff who do battle for patients every day

Abbreviations and Websites

5YFV Five Year Forward View, http://www.england.nhs.uk/wp-content/uploads/2014/10/5yfv-web.pdf.

A&E Accident & Emergency.

AQP Any Qualified Provider.

BMA British Medical Association, http://bma.org.uk/.

BMJ *British Medical Journal,* http://www.bmj.com/.

BUPA British United Provident Association, http://www.bupa.co.uk/.

CCG Clinical Commissioning Groups, (Commissioners), http://www.england.nhs.uk. http://www.nhs.uk/Service-Search/Clinical-Commissioning-Group/LocationSearch/1.

CCP Co-operation and Competition Panel (Monitor): https://www.gov.uk/government/groups/co-operation-and-competition-clinical-reference-group. https://www.gov.uk/government/groups/co-operation-and-competition-economics-reference-group.

CHC Community Health Councils, abolished in England in 2003; they continue to work in Wales, http://www.wales.nhs.uk sitesplus/899/home.

CHPI Centre for Health and the Public Interest, http://chpi.org.uk/.

Clause 119 (HSC Bill) http://www.bbc.co.uk/news/health-26531807.

Commissioning Support Unit (CSU) http://www.england.nhs.uk/resources/css/.

CSIG Commissioning Support Industry Group private interests: e.g. UnitedHealth.

CQC Care Quality Commission, http://www.cqc.org.uk/.

DHA District Health Authority – no longer exists in England.

DoH Department of Health, https://www.gov.uk/government/organisations/department-of-health.

ED Emergency Department.

FoI Freedom of Information (Act), http://www.legislation.gov.uk/ukpga/2000/36/contents.

FT Foundation Trust, http://www.nhsproviders.org/home/.

GMC General Medical Council, http://www.gmc-uk.org/.

Healthwatch http://www.healthwatch.co.uk/find-local-healthwatch.

HSCIC Health and Social Care Information Centre, http://www.hscic.gov.uk/.

HSC Health and Social Care Bill or Act 2012, http://www.legislation.gov.uk/ukpga/2012/7/contents.

HSJ *Health Service Journal, http://*www.hsj.co.uk.

HWBs Health & Wellbeing Board (directory), http://www.kingsfund.org.uk/projects/health-and-wellbeing-boards/hwb-map.

IRP Independent Reconfiguration Panel, https://www.gov.uk/government/organisations/independent-reconfiguration-panel.

ISTC Independent Sector Treatment Centre.

ITU Intensive Therapy/Treatment Unit.

LATs Local area teams, http://www.nhs.uk/servicedirectories/Pages/AreaTeamListing.aspx.

Monitor https://www.gov.uk/government/publications/about-monitor-an-introduction-to-our-role.

MHRA Medicines & Healthcare products Regulatory Agency, http://www.mhra.gov.uk.

NAO National Audit Office, http://www.nao.org.uk/.

NHSCC NHS Clinical Commissioners, http://www.nhscc.org/.

NHS Confederation http://www.nhsconfed.org/.

NHSE NHS England, http://www.england.nhs.uk.

NHS Support Federation http://www.nhscampaign.org/.

NICE National Institute for Health and Clinical Excellence, http://www.nice.org.uk/

Nuffield Trust http://www.nuffieldtrust.org.uk/.

OOH Out of Hours.

PCTs Primary Care Trusts, now replaced by Clinical Commissioning Group.

PFI Private Finance Initiative.

PPI Private Patient Income.

RCN Royal College of Nurses, http://www.rcn.org.uk.

RCGP Royal College of General Practitioners, http://www.rcgp.org.uk.

Section 75 Regulations http://www.legislation.gov.uk/ukpga/2012/7/
section/75/enacted.

SHA Strategic health authorities, abolished in 2013.

SPT Strategic Project Team, http://www.thestrategicprojectsteam.
co.uk.

TDA Trust Development Authority, http://www.ntda.nhs.uk/.

TSA Trust Special Advisor, Trust Special Administrator.

TTIP Transatlantic Trade and Investment Partnership.

TUPE Transfer of Undertakings (Protection of Employment).

UCC Urgent Care Centre.

UH UnitedHealthcare, http://www.uhc.com/.

UNISON Public service trade union, http://www.unison.org.uk.

UNITE Britain's biggest union with 1.42 million in every type of
workplace.
http://www.unitetheunion.org/.

WHO World Health Organisation.

An announcement has been made that hundreds of government
websites will be moving to the gov.uk website https://www.gov.uk.

Foreword

HARRY SMITH

Over ninety years have passed since I was born in the barbarous year of 1923 in the coalmining community of Barnsley. As the light fades on my life, I am drawn towards the narrow cobbled streets of my early life that were fraught with poverty and sickness. Back then existence was a hard scrabble battle for many Britons because we lived in a primitive era when there was no NHS and good health care was a privilege that only the rich could afford.

In the winter of my years, I don't reflect upon my boyhood with nostalgia. It's impossible since I learned too early in my days that life for those who can't access a doctor or medicine due to financial circumstances can be a brief and sad affair. You see, in 1926 when I was a small lad my sister Marion contracted TB and died in a workhouse infirmary because my dad, who had worked as a miner since the age of twelve, was too poor to provide medical care for his daughter on a working-class salary.

Tragically during my childhood in the early twentieth century thousands met their end like Marion. I can even remember as a boy hearing the piercing cries from open windows on our street of people dying from cancer who didn't have the dosh to buy morphine to ease their passage from life. To this day, I am haunted by the inhuman manner in which my sister's illness was treated or how the society of my youth believed that only the well-to-do or well-connected deserved medical care.

That is why after the brutality of the Second World War my generation of ordinary people demanded that our nation create the NHS. We knew it was our only hope of making life better for ourselves, our parents and our children.

The people of my generation sacrificed so much during the Great Depression and through the Second World War and the NHS became our peacetime dividend. The creation of the NHS was also our solemn pledge to future generations that we would be a civilized nation that would treat all citizens as worthy of care and compassion. The NHS is for me as great as Magna Carta because it freed millions from the tyranny of sickness and poverty to move forward and lead productive lives. We must remember that the NHS is as essential to our nation's well-being as the armed forces are to protect us from foreign threats.

It is why today we ordinary citizens must be vigilant against governments and corporate interests that seek to dilute the NHS's ability to deliver health care to all its citizens through privatisation. I am one of the last remaining people that can remember the cruelty of life before the NHS, and I can assure you that it is essential for Britain's prosperity and social well-being that my past doesn't become your future.

Introduction

MARTIN McKEE

How did we ever let it happen? When the then Health and Social Care Bill was passing through parliament (or perhaps one should describe it as drifting, pausing on occasions for a rest, as it is now clear that the attention of the parliamentarians who were meant to scrutinise it was elsewhere), I used the pages of the *British Medical Journal* to ask whether anyone actually understood what the government was hoping to achieve.[1] The Secretary of State's response was not reassuring, suggesting confusion even at the highest levels of government.[2]

Parliamentary draughtsmen are not renowned for the quality of their prose, so they could be forgiven for some of the more turgid stylistic aspects of the Bill. What they are supposed to be good at, however, is rendering complex and often contradictory intentions into clear, explicit, and unambiguous rules. In this case, they failed abysmally. Yet the fault was not theirs. They had been given the impossible task of creating order out of chaos. The result, as has now become abundantly clear, is an Act that is in many respects incomprehensible, frequently contradictory, and causing those who must implement it to scratch their heads in bemusement as they struggle to decide whether what they are doing is even legal, let alone sensible.[3]

In fairness, this reflects the weaknesses of the British system of government, where there are few if any checks on the executive. As long as a prime minister can ensure a majority in parliament (which is rarely difficult given systems of patronage and the dark arts of the whip's office) he or she can ensure the passage of any legislation, no matter how flawed it is. Some legislation has perplexed those charged with implementing it; for example, Lord Justice Rose described the Criminal Justice Act of 2003 Act as 'at best, obscure and, at worst, impenetrable'[4] and in a subsequent case, when faced with the same Act, concluded that

> The most inviting course for this Court to follow would be for its members, having shaken their heads in despair to hold up their hands and say "the Holy Grail of rational interpretation is impossible to find". But it is not for us to desert our judicial duty, however lamentably others have legislated.[5]

As Anthony King and Ivor Crewe note, in their book *The Blunders of our Governments*,[6] there are many other examples of how successive British governments can introduce policies that make things worse, often at great expense. These include Individual Learning Accounts, which despite numerous warnings were an open invitation to organised criminals to extract money from the government, numerous failed information technology (IT) schemes, which had many of the same features, although that time with the IT companies extracting the money. They identify several factors. One is the almost complete disconnect between ministers and civil servants on the one hand and the general public on the other. Another is a form of groupthink, whereby dissenting opinions are either suppressed or ignored. This happens at all legislative stages. Nigel Lawson is said to have missed a crucial meeting on the Poll Tax because he could not imagine that any of his cabinet colleagues would take it seriously. Some commentators have suggested that in such examples there was little or no evidence of the process of parliamentary scrutiny actually fixing any of the problems with policies and legislation.[6] Looked at from this perspective, the 2012 Health and Social Care Act is not so unusual. Its importance instead arises from the impact that it has on everyone living in England. Everyone will use the NHS at some point in their life, from birth to death. They expect it to be there when they need it and, unlike the situation in the USA, they take reassurance from the fact that an unexpected illness will not bankrupt them.[7]

So what did happen? This is something that will be discussed for many years, by policy researchers, historians and, especially, by teachers in business schools seeking case studies of policy failures. The full details may not emerge for many years, until there is publication of the minutes of cabinet meetings and ministerial biographies. Yet even now, some things are clear.

The first is that some people did have a very clear idea of what they wanted the Act to do. As we have documented previously.[8] in 1988 Oliver Letwin, now a government minister, published a book entitled *Privatising the world: a study of international privatisation in theory and in practice*. The foreword was written by the prominent Conservative backbench MP John Redwood. They set out a series of goals for the NHS, including establishing it as a trust independent of government, increasing joint ventures between the NHS and the private sector, extending the principle of charging, with individuals being given personal health budgets, or vouchers, that they could top up if needed. However, they recognised that this would be very difficult to achieve politically. As they noted:

> A system of this sort would be fraught with transitional difficulties. And it would be foolhardy to move so far from the present one in a single leap. But need there be just one leap? Might it not, rather, be possible to work slowly from the present system toward a national insurance scheme? One could begin, for example, with the establishment of the NHS as an independent trust, with increased joint ventures between the NHS and the private sector; move on next to use of 'credits' to meet standard charges set by a central NHS funding administration for independently managed hospitals or districts; and only at the last stage create a national health insurance scheme separate from the tax system.[9]

Clearly, many aspects of the Health and Social Care Act would permit such developments.[10] While all previous purchasing bodies, such as Primary Care Trusts, were responsible for the health of a geographically defined population, the new Clinical Commissioning Groups (CCGs) are not. Moreover, this is a change that the government was absolutely insistent upon. The only plausible reason that it held this position so strongly was to allow CCGs to change, in due course, into competing insurers, offering distinctive packages to different groups within the population. One might focus on the young and healthy, including gym membership but excluding care that would be more important to older people. Of course, some form of risk equalisation system would be introduced but, as experience elsewhere shows, those in the health care business are always several steps ahead of the regulators. The process would be aided by the roll-out of personal health budgets. After all, who could argue with the idea that individuals are best placed to know what health services they need, and indeed this may be true for some people with multiple complex problems. However, as experiences with a wide range of financial services and utilities would have predicted and the Dutch experience with personal health budgets has shown, they also provide numerous opportunities for unscrupulous companies to exploit the vulnerable.[11]

Of course, the Act did not spell out this option. Indeed, it did not spell out very much at all, despite its several hundred pages. Rather, it was worded in a way that would allow such a scenario to develop, along with many others. Thus, its supporters could portray it as a minimal change from the status quo, strengthening the role of the general practitioner, while its critics could equally argue that it would usher in change on a massive scale. Indeed, those critics who were not reassured by ministerial platitudes noted the contradiction between what they were saying and the comment of the NHS Chief Executive that the reforms were so large 'you could see them from space'.

And this is where one of the main difficulties lay. It is very difficult to write legislation in clear English when you are trying to conceal what you are really seeking to achieve. It is even more difficult when ministers draw on Lewis Carroll for their inspiration, failing to realise that *Alice through the Looking Glass* was in many respects an allegory and was certainly not intended as an instruction manual for government. We are expected to laugh at Humpty Dumpty's argument that when he used a word 'it means just what I choose it to mean' and not emulate him.[12] Consequently, despite a convincing argument that what was being proposed actually met all the accepted definitions of privatisation,[13] somehow this word was redefined by ministers to ignore whether health services were delivered by a public or a private provider.

This then poses a problem with implementation. Although diligent observers, sadly outside rather than inside parliament, could spot the problems, the more gullible could be reassured by bland ministerial statements that the sceptics simply did not understand the words that were used. At times, as with the Section 75 competition regulations, the dominant message seemed to be that a true understanding was impossible to those outside the priestly class of ministers and their advisors and that any fears were misplaced.[14] Echoing Voltaire's Dr Pangloss, all would be for the best in the best of all possible worlds.[15] Consequently, many front line workers took these statements at face value, accepting the view that little had really changed. All that the new Act did was to make some minor changes to give the NHS some more freedom from government and give general practitioners a greater role in deciding what services would be provided. The Act emphatically did not promote privatisation, we were told. And to the extent that there would be any increase in non-NHS provision, it would be by friendly social enterprises that were close to their client base but were more flexible than traditional NHS providers in meeting their changing needs. Inevitably, it came as a surprise to many to learn that what they thought were core NHS services were instead being transferred to large international corporations, such as Serco and G4S, a process that continued even after an investigation was launched into whether they had defrauded the Home Office on offender management contracts[16] and after the latter had spectacularly mismanaged security at the London

Olympics.

There is, however, a problem with this model. These large corporations work in many different sectors, from health care, to prisons, to railways, and to the management of London's congestion zone. Their fundamental concern is the bottom line. Where can they make the largest return on investment? And they are slowly realising that this is not in health, with Serco withdrawing from the health market in the United Kingdom.[17] Their entry into the market was predicated on an idea that there was massive waste, with gross overstaffing and overpaid workers. They were able to succeed to some extent in cutting salaries, thereby transferring the cost of employing people to the taxpayer who would top up their salaries in work benefits. But they were less successful in cutting numbers and reducing skill levels. Health care is a labour intensive sector and one in which skills matter. One scandal after another unfolded and it became clear that they were suffering severe reputational risk that would compromise their ability to win contracts in other sectors and other countries.[18-20] They have also realised that the contradictions within the Act, and the resulting confusion, create further barriers to profitability.[21] Instead, they have been focusing on areas where this is not a problem, such as prisons and Australian asylum detention centres where the clients are in no position to complain and can, ideally, be left to look after themselves without the inconvenience of having to pay them.[22]

In British politics it is very rare for politicians to be held accountable for their failures. Indeed, the few cases where this has happened tend to have involved military debacles, such as Churchill at Gallipoli, Chamberlain at Narvik, or Blair in Iraq. In these cases, the scale of the disaster was obvious almost at once and could not be concealed. The Health and Social Care Act is more complicated. It is too easy to lay the blame on other factors, such as the economic crisis (temporarily ignoring the role that the current government has played in making it worse)[23] or an aging and more demanding population. It is also easy to dictate the narrative, especially when most of the major newspapers support one of the parties that implemented the Act. In their excellent book *NHS SOS*,[24] Jacky Davis and Raymond Tallis took the arguments used to justify both the Health and Social Care Act and the legislation enacted by the previous Labour government that paved the way for it and subjected them to the critical examination that our parliamentarians should have done but failed to do. They demonstrated clearly the existential threat that the NHS is facing. Although he subsequently claimed that his words were misinterpreted, in 2004 Oliver Letwin was reported to have said that the NHS would not exist within five years of a Conservative victory.[25] Writing in winter 2014, it seems that he will be proven wrong, but only just. The combination of austerity, transitional costs, and organisational chaos mean that the NHS is suffering almost unprecedented pressures.[26] Waiting times in emergency departments are at the highest level since records began. Morale among health workers is at rock bottom after four years of pay freezes and, in some areas, general practice is nearing collapse. What is to be done?

In this new book, Jacky Davis, joined by John Lister and David Wrigley, look at the continuing threats to the NHS and demolish the myths that have been widely promulgated by those who seek to undermine it. In Chapter 1 they set the scene, reminding us of the broad sweep of events since the passage of the Health and Social Care Act. They warn of the dangers posed by the Trans-Atlantic Trade and Investment Partnership (TTIP) to the provision of all public services, explaining why reassurances to the contrary are at best misinformed and at worst disingenuous.[27]

In Chapter 2 they tackle the claim that 'The NHS can't go on like this'. They remind us that, until the recent reforms, the NHS enjoyed record approval ratings. Historically underfunded compared with health systems in other industrialised countries, the injection of funds after 1999 was followed by sustained improvement in outcomes[28] and it now consistently achieves some of the highest scores in international comparisons of health systems.[29] The argument that an ageing population will render the NHS unsustainable ignores the simple fact that the costs of care are concentrated in the last few months of life, whenever that occurs.[30] Moreover, recent research has shown convincingly that adequate investment in health is actually a driver of economic growth, not as is often suggested, a drag on it.[31-32] It is not that we cannot afford the NHS. Rather, we cannot afford to do without it.

Chapter 3 addresses the myth of choice and competition in health care. Fifty years ago, Kenneth Arrow, a Nobel laureate in economics, showed why markets do not work in health care.[33] Sadly, despite the success of the United States in proving him correct, many commentators are unable, or more likely unwilling, to understand this. As Upton Sinclair famously noted, 'it is difficult to get a man to understand something when his salary depends on his not understanding it'.[34] The reality, as is now becoming apparent in England, is that providers are choosing patients and not the other way round.

Chapter 4 challenges the argument central to the recent reforms that general practitioners will be in the driving seat. In practice, many are walking away from the new commissioning groups, disillusioned by the gap between what was promised and the reality, shocked by some of the more blatant conflicts of interest, and reluctant to accept blame for the inevitable rationing as budgets come under pressure.

Chapter 5 examines the argument that the reformed NHS will be cheaper and have less bureaucracy, showing the enormous costs of compulsory tendering, both for purchasers and providers. Chapter 6 questions whether the reforms deliver on the promise to give more power to local people. As became clear in Lewisham, when local people objected to the downgrading of their local hospital they struggled to be heard and had to take the Secretary of State to court to ensure that he would listen.[35]

Chapter 7 discusses the increasing secrecy of decision making in the NHS, as millions of pounds are disbursed under contracts that are deemed 'commercial in confidence'. It also explores the consequences of freeing the Secretary of State from the requirement to account to parliament for the operations of the NHS.

Chapter 8 tests the claims made for the purported efficiency of the private sector and finds them wanting, while Chapter 9 asks whether the NHS really is being privatised. Government ministers claim they are not, pointing to the still low share of total spending on private providers while ignoring the direction of travel and how, even in the most market-oriented system, the USA, the private sector only wants those parts from which it can make profits, leaving the public sector to pick up the rest.

The book concludes by looking to the future. Chapter 10 considers commercial interests, cuts, closures and 'reconfiguration'. Chapter 11 peers behind the curtain to reveal things they don't want us to know about the dense network of conflicting interests promoting the market in health care.

For the first time this book brings together the evidence of how recent policies have undermined the NHS. It concludes with a challenge to us all. Crucial decisions will have to be made in the months ahead that will have profound consequences for the survival of the NHS. They include those that readers of this book will make in May 2015 as they cast their ballots, those that political parties will make as they write their manifestos, and those that health workers must make as they seek to preserve the health system that, despite its underfunding, remains among the best in the world.

1

Setting the scene

I don't know how much any of you realise that with the Lansley act we pretty much gave away control of the NHS, which means that the thing that most people talk about in terms of health [the NHS] ... we have some important strategic mechanisms but we don't really have day-to-day control.

Jane Ellison MP, Tory public health minister, June 2014

It's hard to believe, but it was not so long ago that the Conservative Party was saying – 'We'll cut the deficit, not the NHS'. Cameron promised there would be no more 'top-down reorganisation' of the NHS and pledged to halt further closures of Accident & Emergency and maternity units. Before the election of 2010 Conservatives were touring the country challenging Labour's record on the NHS, promising year by year increases in NHS spending in real terms.

All of those promises were worthless. The Tories – kept in office by servile Liberal Democrats – have cut public spending, but they have not, as promised, cut the deficit. Indeed even stiffer cutbacks to public sector budgets are required in the next parliament.[1] They have effectively frozen NHS spending, with increases only microscopically higher than inflation, in the meanest five years for funding increases since the NHS was established in 1948.

This funding squeeze has also ensured that the 'moratorium' on closures of A&E and maternity units so proudly announced by Andrew Lansley in the summer of

2010 had become ancient history by the autumn of the same year. The *Daily Telegraph*[2] now calculates that some 66 A&E and maternity units have been closed or downgraded since 2010, or are still under threat.

To make matters worse Cameron's government has forced through the biggest top-down reorganisation in the history of the NHS, with a piece of legislation longer and more complex than the 1946 Act that took hospitals into public ownership and established the NHS as a ground-breaking, integrated public service free to all at point of use, and funded from general taxation.

Eviscerating the NHS

Health Secretary Andrew Lansley's White Paper 'Liberating the NHS', published in July 2010, tore up both Tory and Lib Dem manifesto promises and set out plans for the wholesale top-down reorganisation of the NHS. It was followed swiftly by the Health and Social Care Bill, which eventually received the Royal Assent in 2012 and took effect from April 2013.

The Tories' own verdict on the legislation shifted from uncritical support for Lansley's massive and complex 400-page Bill, to uncertainty mixed with dogged determination to force it through during the brief 'listening exercise' in the spring and summer of 2011, which changed little of substance. By February 2012 David Cameron had to deny stubborn rumours that he and other leading Tories wanted Andrew Lansley 'taken out and shot' for his handling of the Bill.[3]

The NHS in England Reorganised

The new Act abolished Primary Care Trusts (PCTs), the local commissioning bodies which held budgets to buy services for their local population. 150 Primary Care Trusts were replaced by 211 new Clinical Commissioning Groups (CCGs), notionally headed by GPs.

Regional planning was abandoned, with the scrapping of Strategic Health Authorities. In place of these public bodies, which met in public and published their board papers, Lansley's Bill established a new NHS Commissioning Board, (which was soon renamed NHS England), with a network of bureaucratic and secretive Local Area Teams reporting upwards to NHS England but not outwards or downwards to local communities and the wider public.

The over-arching responsibility of the Secretary of State to provide universal and comprehensive health services in England was swept away, handing all of the control over to NHS England and a series of regulators. The 100 or so NHS Trusts were to be compelled either to become free-standing foundation trusts, or to merge with or be taken over by established foundation trusts, which are non-profit businesses accountable only to their governors and not to local communities.

Foundation trusts, which had faced strict limits to the amount of private health care they were allowed to undertake, were also allowed to increase this enormously by the lifting of regulations. They would be permitted under the Act to make up to half of their income from non-NHS work – offering them a possible escape from the pressures of frozen budgets, reduced tariff prices for the care they deliver, and from NHS commissioners seeking to divert ever-larger numbers of patients away from hospital care.

3

The NHS market

Section 75 of the Bill – later reinforced by powerful regulations implemented on the eve of the Act coming into force – set out far-reaching requirements for Clinical Commissioning Groups (CCGs) to put services out to competitive tender. The foundation trust regulator, Monitor, was given wide new powers to regulate the NHS as a whole and, in the amended Bill, to enforce both competition and integration of services.

The competition rules brought completely new players into the regime of competition in the NHS: the Competition Commission and the Office of Fair Trading, both since superseded by the Competition and Markets Authority, began ruling on mergers of trusts,[4] and obstructing collaboration between trusts to improve patient care[5] – on the grounds that it impeded competition.

EU competition law has also become a factor, with its insistence on a so-called 'right to provide' which allows companies to force the opening up of public services to competition. More recently the controversial Transatlantic Trade and Investment Partnership – being negotiated between the EU and the US administration, with full support from the British government, and leading members of the Parliamentary Labour Party – has also become a potential factor. It may create major obstacles to bringing privatised services back into public ownership and control.[6]

Labour's opposition to Lansley's Health and Social Care Bill was weak at first. The party mounted no significant campaign outside Parliament. The unions, following suit, were also slow to develop any real campaign. In bizarre fashion the most influential early opposition to Lansley's Bill came from the Tories' coalition partners, in particular from LibDem rank-and-file party members. At their spring conference in

2011 they were manoeuvred out of a vote that could have overturned Liberal Democrat support for the Bill.

The LibDem reservations were enough to force Cameron into a highly unorthodox 'pause' in the process of legislation in late spring and early summer of 2011. The tame former GP leader Professor Steve Field was brought in to head up an NHS Future Forum in a 'listening exercise' which managed to avoid listening to any significant numbers of the general public or campaigners. After the 'pause' it was back to business as usual. The huge and complex Bill, barely altered, ground on through the Commons, where it seems that among the many Tories who voted for it without understanding it was Jeremy Hunt, later to be named as Lansley's successor as Health Secretary.[7]

GPs reject Lansley plan

One group who remained unconvinced from beginning to end were GPs – whose main voice challenging the Bill was not the docile, ambivalent BMA but the Royal College of General Practitioners. Each RCGP poll showed a large majority of those allegedly empowered by the Bill declaring their opposition to it. Early in 2012, recognising this huge credibility gap, Lansley issued a letter to all GPs, which appeared to reassure them that – contrary to all but ministers' reading of the Bill – there would be no requirement on CCGs to privatise or put services out to tender (see Chapter 4). It was only at this stage that Labour – with Andy Burnham now leading the way as shadow health secretary – began to wage a belated, but largely inward-looking campaign against the Act. The TUC unions threw resources into a big, lively but again belated rally in Westminster Central Hall, in March 2012, but it was too little, too late.

The LibDem spring conference in 2012 saw the definitive collapse of any real opposition as another critical motion was blocked by party leaders, terrified that a breach in the coalition would trigger an early election. Shirley Williams, the party's proclaimed standard-bearer, meekly accepted Tory assurances and threw in the towel, giving her support for the Bill, thus ensuring it passed the Lords on the strength of LibDem votes. LibDem votes also carried the controversial Regulations that gave real teeth to Section 75 of the Act. Among other things the Regulations set out the few, wholly exceptional circumstances in which CCGs might be excused from putting services out to tender.

The effects of the Health and Social Care Act

The consequences of this wholesale reorganisation of the National Health Service via the Health and Social Care Act are already starting to make themselves felt. Organisational upheaval, the fragmentation of services and organisations due to new requirements for services to be put out to tender, and the underlying, worsening financial squeeze on the NHS (driven by the Cameron government's commitment to austerity and cuts in public spending until at least 2021) are combining to push the system ever further into crisis.

There are indications that even the Tories themselves, having pushed the Act through, are now beginning to view this huge piece of complex legislation as a major mistake, with David Cameron reportedly admitting he did not know what it entailed, even when he took personal charge of getting it onto the statute book.[8] Other Tories have been equally baffled or critical of the Act and its outcome. Tory public health minister Jane Ellison (as quoted above) was recorded in June 2014 telling a Tory Reform Group meeting that as a result of the Act the government had effectively given away day-to-day control of the NHS.[9] Clause 1 of the Act was the key factor in giving away control, abolishing as it did the duty of the Secretary of State to provide universal and comprehensive services in England.

Section 75 of the Act, backed up by wide-ranging additional regulations, focuses on creating a competitive market in health services, and increasingly the contracts offered up are being won by the private sector.[10] Vital cash from NHS budgets is flowing out of the NHS into private companies seeking profits from health care. While the private sector revels in its rising revenues, the money they win in contracts is taken from the limited NHS budget, leaving less for the NHS trusts and services which remain the bedrock and only option for many key services which the private sector sees as risky or unprofitable.

Emergency services and care of the most seriously ill suffer cuts, while managers have to focus their attention on tenders offering the easiest elective and community services to profit-hungry companies seeking to slice out the safest returns. NHS management time and resources which should be concentrated on patient care are increasingly being squandered on complex contractual arrangements and 'commercial' activity,[11] supervised by the regulator Monitor (with its additional powers to enforce competition) and even by the newly-formed Competition and Markets Authority.

NHS England

What has all this done to our NHS? One of the first casualties has been the accountability of the service. The Commons Public Administration Select Committee has raised searching questions over the level of accountability, if any, of the new, all-powerful national commissioning board, known as NHS England, which controls some £95.6bn of NHS funds. Asked what the system of accountability was between the Department of Health and NHS England, the civil servant responsible gave the committee a bafflingly convoluted 300-word answer. At the end of 2014, Bernard Jenkin, Tory chair of the Committee questioned the complex relationship that the Act has established between the Department of Health and NHS England, the 'arm's length' commissioning board.[12]

> Vast amounts of money are involved here, £95.6bn in the case of NHS England alone, and it is simply not acceptable that there is no clarity or clear accountability for that kind of public expenditure … The architecture is not meant to be reminiscent of the film *The Matrix* where doors open on virtual worlds which are insulated from reality and hidden from the public and from those meant to be accountable for them.[13]

NHS England itself is now headed by Simon Stevens, a one-time political advisor to Tony Blair, who then spent ten years in the private sector, working for giant US health insurance corporation UnitedHealth, (where he became Executive Vice President). It is chaired by Professor Sir Malcolm Grant, former provost at University College, London, who has complained of 'meddling' by government ministers in the running of the NHS.[14]

Level playing fields?
NHS England's plans to cut the 'minimum practice income guarantee' which supports GP services in deprived and rural areas produced an angry reaction from hard-pressed GPs

who warned it could trigger substantial numbers of practice closures. Amid street protests led by GPs in East London, NHS England had to retreat, shelving the problem for at least two years. NHS England has also been found in the High Court to have repeatedly departed from the provisions of the HSC Act by imposing changes in primary care services without any mechanism to consult or engage with patients and public in the affected localities.[15]

NHS England has been prone to blunders. It is so isolated and remote from the real world that it has been slow to recognise its mistakes. For example, a formula for commissioning specialist services for the care of offenders with severe mental illness proved to be ill-conceived. It was based on the ostensibly lower daily fee for secure placements charged by some private sector providers, below the cost of delivering the superior and more effective services in specialist NHS Trusts. The result would have been a long-term increase in costs, since the lower levels of therapeutic treatment in the private units would mean that offenders would stay there for far longer, and would be more likely to reoffend after discharge. NHS England had to retreat on this plan – although the problem is still not finally resolved as this chapter is completed.

In October 2014 further fears of NHS England incompetence were provoked by new plans to stop commissioning specialist renal services i.e. dialysis and transplants. NHSE announced a minimal six-week 'consultation' spanning the Christmas period. Thereafter (from April 2015) they looked forward to dumping the problem onto ill-prepared Clinical Commissioning Groups. This move has been roundly condemned by the British Kidney Patient Association as endangering access to care and potentially putting lives at risk.[16]

There is also widespread and growing chaos at the local level. Inexperienced Clinical Commissioning Groups, pressed by the Health and Social Care Act and associated regulations, and often led by a handful of maverick GPs or, from behind the scenes, by management consultants, are drawing up ever more far-reaching and irresponsible plans for contracting out services. Some are doing this regardless of the potential impact on local NHS trusts if the contracts – and the funding – are won by private sector bids.

Already some CCGs are awarding contracts to the private sector for Musculoskeletal (MSK) services, and these potentially destabilise local NHS trauma services and therefore the viability of A&E departments. Elsewhere a variety of other services – care of older people, cancer care, end of life care, and a range of community health services such as community beds, specialist community nursing, community therapy, podiatry, early supported discharge and intermediate care – are being put out to tender, with a combined value of billions over five to ten years. If private sector firms succeed in winning these contracts, they will undermine the viability of dozens of local trusts which provide other vital services to their local communities.

It's all getting out of hand, but it's important to remember that the new drive towards privatisation and fragmentation is not the only aspect of government policy that threatens the future of the NHS. The crisis in the NHS dates back to the great 2008-9 banking crash which heralded the end of a record ten successive years of investment in the NHS from 2000 to 2010, and which has taken five years to come fully to the surface.

It's a crisis which combines the impact of the unprecedented five-year spending freeze (which is driving indebted hospital trusts to rationalise and cut back local services to save money), with a growing fragmentation and dislocation of the newly-reorganised system. The fragmentation certainly began under Tony Blair's Labour government, but it has been vastly accelerated and deepened by the impact of the Health and Social Care Act.

The long freeze

The driving force in this latest crisis has been the Tory-led coalition government, which has cynically seized upon the pretext of the economic dislocation triggered by the banking crash as justification for imposing its neoliberal austerity policies on the NHS. Of course Cameron and his ministers energetically deny this, and profess their total commitment to the NHS and its values. When challenged on the inadequate level of funding, along with lengthening waiting times and queues for treatment and the rising debts of local NHS and foundation trusts, David Cameron insists the government has put 'an extra £12.5bn' into the NHS since it took office. Over five years, that works out roughly £2.5bn per year – just a fraction above inflation, but increasingly falling short of the rising costs of meeting the health needs of a growing population.

Tory chancellor George Osborne has planned for this freeze to continue at least until 2021. However, almost all experts not on the government payroll are agreed that this would result in a massive potential £30bn gap between NHS income and costs of delivering services. Despite the Tory rhetoric before and since, the election of 2010 brought not only a change of government, but the start of a new era of frozen real terms budgets, which will have risen by a total of just 0.1 per cent above general inflation in five years.[17]

The same period has seen a significant rise in the total population, and in numbers of older people, who tend to make greater demands on the NHS. The Institute for Fiscal Studies estimates that if the spending freeze is maintained it could cut age-related per capita spending on the NHS by 9.1 per cent from 2010 to 2019.[18] Other cost pressures, including the bill for new drugs and techniques, have continued to mount up. Estimates of the rising cost pressures vary – but it is commonly assumed that increases in spending above inflation of 3-4 per cent each year are needed to maintain and grow services and maintain performance.

Up to the arrival of the coalition, spending had risen on average just over 4 per cent a year since the NHS was formed (although this average is itself inflated by Labour's big spending increases from 2000 to 2010).[19] The NHS budget had never before been frozen for any sustained length of time. We are in unexplored waters.

On top of the regular pressures there have been costly pressures from ministers, too. Health Secretary Jeremy Hunt has insisted that NHS trusts – regardless of financial pressures – must increase nurse and other staffing levels to comply with the recommendations of the Francis Report on the catastrophic failures of care at Mid Staffordshire Hospitals from 2005-2008.[20] As a result thousands more nurses have been recruited, leaving many trusts facing deep deficits, while the Care Quality Commission is warning that more than three quarters of trusts are failing to deliver adequate safety for patients.[21] Estimates in the McKinsey report[22] made back in 2009 suggest that the cumulative gap in resources for the NHS would reach a total of £20bn by

2015. The report, commissioned by then Health Secretary Alan Johnson, outlined ideas (many of them impractical) for 'cost savings'. Despite being officially disavowed both by the Labour government that commissioned it and by the Tories, who denounced it in opposition and then published it once elected – these ideas have shaped subsequent plans of trust boards and local commissioners for 'cost savings'.

Also in 2009, amid growing concern over the need for a mechanism to force through unpopular local decisions to close hospitals that failed in the new, emerging competitive 'market' for health care, Labour tweaked its 2006 legislation to create the 'Unsustainable Provider Regime',[23] which has now been tweaked again by Jeremy Hunt, seeking even more draconian powers in the aftermath of his bruising defeat over cuts at Lewisham Hospital (see Chapter 10).

The coalition has outlined financial plans that include a continued freeze on NHS budgets running right up to 2020, while other sectors of public spending face further cuts. Even in the 'ring-fenced' NHS the proposals would open up an unprecedented decade of standstill funding, culminating in what forecasters – including the Nuffield Trust, King's Fund, Monitor, NHS England and its chief executive Simon Stevens[24] – have calculated as *another* £30bn gap in spending over the five years from 2015. To give some idea of the scale of the problem, had Labour in 2000 implemented a similar freeze rather than their big increases in spending up to 2010, England's NHS budget would now be just £75bn per year – almost 30 per cent lower than the current £105bn.

So far the impact of the squeeze on spending has been to a large extent concealed by a disproportionate cut in the real salaries of over one million NHS staff covered by the 'Agenda for Change' pay structure. Pay for these staff has either been frozen or risen well below inflation each year since 2009, bringing real terms reductions in pay of upwards of 12 per cent since 2010 for lower paid staff, and 16 per cent or more for nurses and professionals above Band 5 on the pay scale. But all observers of the unfolding situation are now warning that the pay cuts cannot go on for ever, and that the additional £30bn cuts, at a time when most trusts are already mired in deficits, simply cannot be absorbed without doing serious damage to the NHS. The NHS Confederation has pointed out that one consequence could be reopening the question of charging patients to see GPs or for stays in hospital.[25]

NHS funding – barking up the wrong tree

The King's Fund's Barker Commission[26] began from the assumption that that no government party would raise taxes to spend enough to protect the NHS. The Commission drew up a list of unappealing options to raise money in less progressive ways, including wider imposition of prescription charges, and a series of taxes and costs for those over retirement age. The more right-wing 'think tanks' have of course wheeled back out their vintage plans to impose charges for treatment, for a £10 per head annual 'membership fee' for the NHS, or to drive those who can afford it towards private health insurance.[27]

As the commentator Roy Lilley has observed, whether health funding comes from one pocket through charges for treatment or drugs, or from the other pocket through taxes, it is 'the same trousers'. Health spending has to go up, or services have to be cut. But of course if the extra is raised through charges, the burden of cost falls least fairly and sustainably on individuals (often the very young, very old or the poor) who are sick and obliged to pay, while those who are not sick make no contribution.

The 2014 party conferences, at which Labour, Tories and Lib Dems largely set out their stalls for the next election, saw each party timidly sidestepping any commitment to restore the purchasing power of the NHS or substantially break from the continued decline in real terms funding proposed by the coalition until at least 2020. Labour promised a 'Time to Care Fund' of £2.5bn per year – but to be funded through taxes on 'mansions' worth more than £2m, hedge funds and tobacco industry profits – which may not yield any revenue until 2017.[28] The Lib Dems offered an even more feeble injection of £1bn in 2016 and again in 2017, while the Tories stuck to their misleading claim to be 'increasing NHS funding' and again pledged to 'ring-fence' the NHS budget, suggesting at best a microscopic percentage above inflation up to 2020.

None of these policies offers any hope for sustaining current levels of service to the end of the decade, meaning that whichever party wins the election in 2015 will be plunged almost immediately into a chaos of cuts and closures, in which (as we have seen in every previous such period) opportunist individual ministers and MPs inevitably break ranks with their government to side with local campaigners.

Tender spots

The scenario of recent cuts is further complicated by the menacing tide of competitive tendering and privatisation leading to increased fragmentation.

The drive towards privatisation has been accelerated and intensified by the Tory-led coalition. By contrast, immediately prior to the 2010 election, Andy Burnham, who had taken over as Secretary of State from Alan Johnson in June 2009, had moved swiftly to end the pressure for community health services to be opened up for tenders from 'any willing provider' that had been initiated as part of Labour's plans under Patricia Hewitt, and driven forward by Johnson.

Instead, to the fury of Blairites in his own party, along with the private sector and some of the voluntary sector organisations that were queuing up for NHS contracts, Burnham ruled that the NHS should be the 'preferred provider'.[29] This left the purchaser/provider split and the framework of a competitive market intact. This was strenuously challenged, but Burnham managed to hold the line until the election, after which the new Health Secretary, Andrew Lansley, within weeks unfurled plans to open up not just community health services but many other parts of the NHS to any willing provider – later grudgingly and ambiguously amended in the Health and Social Care Bill to 'any qualified provider'.

PFI – Profits for Industry

There is also a growing threat to the future of services in and around some of the country's newest hospitals. The Private Finance Initiative's (PFI) expensive long-term contracts have often resulted in rising costs, and in inflated and unaffordable financial burdens. The Royal Assent to the Health and Social Care Act in April 2012 shifted attention to other aspects of the growing crisis in the NHS. One of these was the lingering bitter legacy of the hospital developments financed at inflated costs through PFI in deals signed by the Labour government from 1997.

The PFI originated as a Tory policy in the early 1990s. According to *Guardian* financial columnist Larry Elliott, the PFI was 'a scam':

Of all the scams pulled by the Conservatives in 18 years of power – and there were plenty – the Private Finance

Initiative was perhaps the most blatant. ... If ever a piece of ideological baggage cried out to be dumped on day one of a Labour government it was PFI.[30]

Labour had originally opposed it. Margaret Beckett, shadow health secretary in 1995, summed up what had become a common line from Labour when she told the *Health Service Journal*: 'As far as I am concerned PFI is totally unacceptable. It is the thin end of the wedge of privatisation.'[31] But in the final months of John Major's Tory government, Tony Blair's team abruptly ditched the party's stance of opposition and in the summer of 1996 Shadow Treasury minister Mike O'Brien announced the new policy: 'This idea must not be allowed to fail. Labour has a clear programme to rescue PFI.'[32]

By the spring of 1998, PFI had become: 'A key part of the (Labour) Government's 10 year modernisation programme for the health service.'[33] Thus after years of rejecting PFI as a step towards privatisation, it was inserted into Labour's 1997 manifesto, with the pledge to 'sort out' the idea of PFI and make it work.[34] For the NHS this was done by pushing through a short Bill in 1997 making a far-reaching commitment that the Secretary of State would act as guarantor for PFI schemes, undertaking to pick up any outstanding costs if an NHS Trust went broke and was no longer able to pay.[35] This undertaking removed any real risk from private investors, and the first wave of schemes began to be signed off in the first few years of the Blair government, while Tory cash limits still prevailed.

The first PFI hospital opened in 2000. It was seen as a magical way of securing new capital investment while deferring the costs and spreading them over thirty years or more. Almost all of the earliest schemes combined capital investment in the building with long-term contracts for the provision of non-clinical support services (cleaning, catering, porters, maintenance, and security). The right to franchise retail outlets and car parking revenues were also generally all rolled up into complex contracts, with a single 'unitary charge' to be paid by the NHS trust, rising each year by 2.5 per cent or inflation, whichever was the higher. The NHS Trust was left in charge only of budgets for clinical services and staff – everything else was in effect handed over to the PFI 'partner'.

Although in hindsight many of the first-wave schemes appear to be small in value (many new hospitals costing around £100m or even less), a number of them have turned out to be extremely costly over the lifetime of the contract. Many trusts found that the legally-binding charges consumed an unaffordable share of their overall income, with increasingly serious consequences. The problem has been exacerbated in the last few years by the freeze on NHS funding, by additional inflation, and by subsequent schemes for building a number of far more expensive new PFI hospitals, with really hefty annual charges which have caused major problems for some trusts.

The latest overall figures published on the Treasury website show £11.6bn worth of NHS schemes in England are set to cost almost £80bn over the lifetime of their contracts, averaging seven times the capital cost (although some first wave trusts are costing far more). And while the unitary charge payments per year are now just 2 per cent of NHS spending (around £2bn), some trusts are having to fork out a far higher share of their budget for extortionate schemes.

The Costs of PFI: Amersham, Coventry, etc.

Amersham Hospital, a £45m development, is costing 11.6 times the capital cost: the Trust has already paid almost five times the cost, and still has 15 years left to pay. Calderdale has already paid more than four times the original cost, but will wind up paying the cost 12 times over. The 970-bed £158m Norfolk & Norwich Hospital, too small and struggling from day one, has also already paid back four times the capital cost, but has another £2.2bn to pay – coming out at 14.7 times the original investment.

Among the more recent big PFIs which are costing above the average are Coventry's £379m University Hospital, which has so far paid back more than double the investment, but has another £3.3bn left to pay: and St Helens & Knowsley, where a £338m hospital will cost £3.8bn under PFI.

Even PFI contracts involving total payments on or below the average seven-fold can involve costs that are simply unaffordable. The Sherwood Forest Foundation Trust's new King's Mill Hospital and related projects cost £326m and will cost a relatively modest £2.4bn, just above the average 7:1 ratio: but the Trust is not a large one, and the unitary charge payments come out at an unsustainable 16 per cent of the trust's revenue.[36]

In Peterborough, where a ridiculous £320m contract was signed off by the Board in defiance of a warning letter from Monitor, the £40m-plus payments are an unmanageable 20 per cent of the Trust's revenue. As a result the new hospital has had to be propped up with Department of Health subsidies since it opened, while costly teams of management consultants have tried in vain to resolve the impossible situation of an unaffordable hospital serving a large catchment that is 35 miles from its nearest equivalent, and 25 miles from the nearest district hospital, Hinchingbrooke.[37]

The first PFI bankruptcy

In 2012 the impact of PFI came dramatically to the fore with the combined crises of two South East London first wave PFIs, the Queen Elizabeth Hospital in Woolwich, and the Princess Royal Hospital in Orpington. These had been merged into the giant, debt-ridden South London Healthcare Trust, bringing their cumulative debts and soaring costs with them. The two hospitals had cost a total of £214m to build, but are set to cost the NHS and taxpayer £2.6bn to repay over thirty years. By the time Secretary of State Andrew Lansley invoked the 'unsustainable provider regime' in July 2012 the South London Healthcare Trust had a cumulative deficit of £207m.[38]

Interestingly, the draconian powers wielded by the Trust Special Administrator (TSA) who was brought in to propose a way forward were not deployed to challenge or force any renegotiation of the disastrous PFI contracts, which even the TSA admitted saddled the Trust with capital costs far above the NHS average. In fact all the concessions were made on behalf of the NHS; the plans drawn up included not only writing off the back debts, but a hefty annual subsidy to underwrite some of the excess cost of each scheme until the contracts are paid off – bringing the bail-out cost to more than £600m.

Of course, little attention centred on this aspect of the crisis, because the TSA, desperate to find some assets to plunder in order to minimise the cost of the bail-out, seized on the idea of closing down and selling off two thirds of the neighbouring, but unrelated, Lewisham Hospital.

This triggered local outrage and a succession of very large protest meetings, lobbies and demonstrations These culminated in a legal challenge mounted jointly by the campaigners and Lewisham council, which early in 2013 overturned this aspect of the TSA proposals, on the grounds that the Administrator, by taking action in an adjacent trust, had exceeded even the sweeping powers he had been given.[39] Once the initial ruling had been upheld on appeal, the petulant response from Jeremy Hunt, Lansley's successor as Secretary of State, was to take steps to prevent any such setback in future by adding two hugely controversial 'hospital closure' clauses to the otherwise unrelated Care Bill then going through Parliament. This means that in future situations, a TSA can make far-reaching cuts in any trust in the vicinity of the 'failing' trust, leaving nobody's services safe.

Lessons from Mid Staffordshire

In February 2013 the headlines were dominated by the publication of the Francis Report[40] which summed up the evidence on the long-running inquiry into events at the Mid Staffordshire Hospitals Foundation Trust in 2005-8. The massive 1100-page Report focused on the catastrophic failure of health care which had been triggered by cutbacks in staffing to save money, and a brutally insensitive management regime at the Trust. The report itself contained some very important points, but ducked many key issues.

- It avoided pinning direct responsibility on any of the senior managers whose indifference, negligence and bullying of staff ensured such appalling lapses from acceptable standards and went on for so long without intervention or investigation.
- It proposed legal obligations on NHS front-line staff to report failures in care, but offered them no protection against managers who respond with bullying and victimisation.
- It failed to address the flawed 'reforms' and the unrealistic

financial targets that had led Mid Staffs management into such desperate actions – and are still forcing similar decisions from NHS managers all over England.

- It argued correctly in the body of the report that 'it was or should have been the directors' primary responsibility to ensure either that they did deliver an acceptable standard of service or, if this was not possible, to say so loudly and clearly, and take whatever steps were necessary to protect their patients'. However the Report's conclusions included no specific recommendation that might ensure this could happen.

Many of the 290 recommendations which the Report did make were ignored or immediately dismissed by the coalition government. However, more recent signs of panic over falling staffing levels suggest a continued uncertainty among ministers over the long-term fallout from the report as they force the pace of cash savings.

Soon after the Francis Report appeared the Unsustainable Provider Regime was again invoked, and a triumvirate comprised of a clinician and two Ernst & Young accountants were appointed as joint Trust Special Administrators tasked with the rundown and closure of Stafford hospital. However, despite all the colossal barrage of negative publicity about the Trust (which by then had a completely new management regime, and was performing far better than most equivalent trusts), the proposed closure drew massive local protests with around 50,000 marching through the town demanding to keep the hospital open, a fight that has continued into the final months of 2014.

CCGs – Cranky Commissioning Groups

As 2013 progressed there were increasing tell-tale signs of the chaos, waste and bureaucracy that would be unleashed by the Health and Social Care Act. In March a detailed *British Medical Journal* study based on Freedom of Information inquiries to the 211 new Clinical Commissioning Groups found that more than a third of the GPs taking seats on the boards had conflicts of interest, in the form of a financial interest in a for-profit private provider from which their CCG could potentially commission services. This proportion was higher among GPs than among the other members of the CCG Boards.[41]

A *Yorkshire Post* investigation exposed the fact that Monitor, about to take on an expanded role in regulating the whole of the NHS, had spent a third of its £19.5m budget in the previous year on consultancy fees for advice from PriceWaterhouseCooper, Deloitte, McKinsey and KPMG.[42]

The summer of 2013 saw the Health and Social Care Act take effect as Cambridgeshire and Peterborough CCGs announced plans to invite tenders to deliver a complex new 'pathway' for Older People's services, with the first shortlist of ten featuring a majority of private-sector-led bids. Neighbouring Bedfordshire CCG soon followed, putting the county's Musculoskeletal (MSK) services up for tender – in which the front-running and eventually successful tender was led by Circle and included Horizon Health Choices, a company owned by almost half the GP practices in Bedfordshire.[43]

While elective and community health services were clearly the focus of the private sector, other parts of the NHS and social care were facing a tightening squeeze. From 2012 onwards it became clear that spending on mental health services, always a poor relation of the wider NHS, but which had been allocated slightly more generous resources in the 2000s, was actually declining for the first time in over a decade.[44] This decline was accelerated in the first year of the CCGs, reinforcing the concerns of mental health staff that GPs and their commissioning support groups did not properly understand or value mental health care but tended to focus only on the provision of 'talking therapies' for those with relatively less severe problems such as depression, while more specialist services and hospital care for those in greatest need was cut back in CCG contracts. During 2013-14 the spotlight fell on the national shortage of specialist Child and Adolescent Mental Health Service beds, with vulnerable young people having to be transported often hundreds of miles for inpatient care.[45]

Ministers, mostly LibDems, have pushed through policies on paper which seem to press for 'parity of esteem' between mental health and other health services,[46] although this is hard to achieve in the context of continued cutbacks in resources, not least in the commissioning decisions of NHS England, which controls specialist budgets.

Cutbacks in acute hospital services remained firmly in the limelight in several areas of London in particular, notably north-west London. Here commissioners had drawn up plans for the biggest ever wave of closures in a single area, with four A&E units due to close, along with virtually all acute services at Ealing and Charing Cross Hospitals. A long and bitter campaign to challenge the plans, which were blithely entitled 'Shaping a Healthier Future' resulted in Ealing council's oversight and scrutiny committee invoking its right to force a decision on the closures from Secretary of State Jeremy Hunt. He in turn brought in the Independent

Reconfiguration Panel, which after some investigation and deliberation gave its stamp of approval to the closures of A&E units at Hammersmith and Central Middlesex Hospitals, but pronounced itself unconvinced by the proposals for alternative services to pick up displaced caseload from Ealing and Charing Cross. The trusts were told to maintain services until more convincing plans had been drawn up and alternative services put in place.[47]

From the end of 2013 into 2014 warnings were beginning to sound over the impact of the continued spending freeze, and CCG plans were becoming even more irresponsible. In the East Midlands 19 CCGs resorted to plans for cuts and closures of existing services in their efforts to cut spending by more than £1bn over the next five years, despite rising populations and even more rapidly growing numbers of older patients with greater health needs.[48]

In Leicestershire, a massively indebted trust borrowed money to open extra beds and meet targets at the same time as the county's CCGs drew up plans to close down hundreds more beds and scale down hospital services. In Lincolnshire, plans to save £105m over five years are focused primarily on making huge savings from cuts in A&E, maternity and paediatrics by 'centralising' on just one site – regardless of the journey times and problems this would pose patients, parents and their visitors. Taking 'care closer to home' to new levels of absurdity, the CCGs regard all of the beds in the homes of the county's 700,000 population as 'community' settings.

In Nottinghamshire, two separate plans aimed for massive cutbacks in hospital treatment, trying to slash not only numbers using A&E but also numbers of emergency admissions, acute hospital bed days, and even to cut referrals to nursing homes by 25 per cent. In North Derbyshire the CCG wants to cut 'avoidable emergency admissions' by 22 per cent – despite the fact that the increase in emergency and elective caseload at nearby hospitals is because patients are being sent there by GPs! In South Derbyshire, where the £300m PFI-burdened Derby Hospitals Trust has been running at a deficit, the CCG plans to save itself money by redirecting patients away from the hospital to 'the community' – despite having no concrete plans to establish the services patients would need. In Northamptonshire, (designated as a 'challenged health economy' seeking huge 'savings' of £276m in health and social care) the Nene CCG is attempting to solve its own financial problems by imposing hefty financial penalties on the struggling Northampton General Hospital Trust for exceeding target numbers for emergency admissions, although the high and rising numbers flow from the CCG's own failure to put any alternative services in place.

CCGs have also been drawing up irresponsible plans to put other services out to tender, potentially jeopardising local trusts: in Staffordshire, contracts for the control of £1.2bn worth of cancer and end of life care have been put out to tender by several CCGs egged on and funded by Macmillan, the cancer support charity.[49] In Cornwall, NHS Kernow has decided to put £75m worth of elective services out to tender – a massive share of the budget of the county's only acute trust,[50] despite the consequences for the Royal Cornwall Hospitals Trust if the contracts are awarded to the private sector.

Utilising another aspect of the HSC Act, some foundation trusts, under severe financial pressures, have cranked up their private work resulting in massive increases of up to 40 per cent in their income from private patients.[51]

Vanishing social care

Social care is facing a massive financial squeeze. Between March 2011 and March 2014 £2.68bn will have been 'saved' by adult social care in England, equivalent to 20 per cent of the budget, according to forecasts by the Association of Directors of Adult Social Services[52] – figures broadly confirmed and underlined by the more recent Age UK report *Care in Crisis*. As a result of the years of cutbacks 87 per cent of councils have so far restricted eligibility for social care to service users with 'substantial' or even more severe needs. This means that those who do receive care tend to be relatively more expensive to support: so a 25 per cent reduction in the number of people supported to live at home in the five years to 2012 brought only a 5 per cent reduction in actual spending.

According to the Audit Commission, a reducing share of adult social care spending is now allocated to older patients, with more going instead to those with learning disabilities and mental health problems. Average spending per resident aged 65 and over was 13 per cent lower in 2012 than in 2010. The percentage cut in spending per head appears even higher because budgets are reducing as numbers of older people increase. The 2013 spending round will lead to a further 10 per cent cut in overall council budgets in 2015/16.[53]

NHS in decline

Since the coalition came into power the previous gains made by the NHS have gone into reverse. Growing pressures on the diminishing hospital services result in increasing and under-funded demand on A&E, the return of lengthening waiting times, and more delays in discharging patients from hospital for lack of suitable support in the community. A recent report in *The Times*[54] shows the decline:

- Since 2010 there has been an increase of a third in the numbers waiting for operations, now 3.3 million.
- Average waits for treatment have lengthened by over 10 per cent.
- There has been a 25 per cent increase in the numbers waiting over 18 weeks and over 26 weeks for outpatient appointments and treatment.
- Cancer treatment targets have been missed for two successive quarters.
- For well over a year A&E departments have been failing to hit targets for treatment within four hours.
- Trolley waits for a bed have almost trebled in the last three years.
- Last minute cancellation of operations last year hit the highest level for nine years.
- Delayed discharge of patients fit enough to leave hospital have hit a new record level.
- 60 per cent of patients have to wait more than 48 hours to see a GP.

Mutual loathing

In the summer of 2014, the Tory-led coalition revived yet another policy initiative that had been first developed by New Labour from 2005 – the promotion of 'social enterprises' or 'mutuals' as a business model for what had formerly been NHS providers – the so-called 'John Lewis' model.

By bizarre coincidence the renewed campaign kicked off at the very point when the most prominent self-proclaimed 'mutual', the private hospital chain Circle, which had famously won a ten-year contract to manage Hinchingbrooke Hospital, wound up the 'partnership' that had appeared to give staff 'shares' equivalent to almost 50 per cent of the company. These Circle shares were always very strange: they paid no dividend, gave no control, and could not be sold. Now they have been scrapped, Circle is simply a Jersey-based company almost entirely owned by hedge fund and city interests, while new shares, equivalent to less than 10 per cent of the company, have been issued on an unclear basis to staff, who still have no real control.

A report by health union UNISON[55] also showed that despite the rhetoric, there is and was NO partnership working at Hinchingbrooke. Circle has refused even to meet the trade unions representing staff at the hospital, and a disastrous NHS staff survey showed relationships between management and staff at Hinchingbrooke are worse than the average for the whole NHS. Out of 28 key findings, Hinchingbrooke came out worse than the NHS average on two thirds (19), and in the lowest 20 per cent of trusts in almost half.[56]

Nonetheless in July 2014 Tory grandee Francis Maude joined with LibDem health minister Norman Lamb and former Blairite minister Hazel Blears to launch a campaign to persuade hard-pressed foundation trusts to float off FTs as mutual/social enterprises.[57] Interestingly the government definition of a public service mutual, according to the literature for the new Pathfinder Programme, is an organisation that 'has spun out of the public sector'.[58]

The truth is that mutuals are no longer part of the NHS: they are non-profit businesses, and their staff are guaranteed none of the benefits of NHS terms and conditions, training schemes, or pensions. These are among the reasons why Labour encountered such stubborn resistance from staff when they attempted to push Community Health Services towards mutual status.[59]

Few staff other than the most senior managers driving the process accepted the absurd claim (recently echoed by Chris Ham of the King's Fund[60]) that mutuals would increase staff engagement, empower them to improve services, or in any way benefit them or their patients. In the few instances where ballots were allowed before frog-marching unwilling staff into these 'partnerships' the votes against were 80-90 per cent or higher. Back in 2006 the first social enterprise to win a substantial contract, Central Surrey Health, had pressed ahead with the bid in the teeth of opposition from 84 per cent of their staff.[61]

The coalition plan to promote mutuals involves putting £1m up front to subsidise the costs of 10 'pathfinder' foundation or NHS trusts in paying for 'bespoke technical, legal and consultancy support' – giving an early foretaste of the increased bureaucratic costs involved if they press ahead and launch as mutuals. It's unlikely to stop at that point. Francis Maude in particular is already looking to mutuals and charities as a less politically damaging way to break up the NHS and other public services.[62] It's clear that even those mutuals that manage to survive will struggle to retain their contracts against predatory private sector bids when they next come up for tender. Mutuals are both a step outside the public sector and a big step on the road to full privatisation.

Crooked path to privatisation

However, this roundabout route to privatisation is another useful reminder that the private sector have not had it all their own way despite the framework of legislation that has been put in place by a privatising, neoliberal government committed to creating a competitive market in health care.

In October 2014 it was announced that the biggest contract

yet put out to tender, the £800m, five-year contract for Older People's services in Cambridgeshire and Peterborough, had been won by the NHS bid, led by Cambridge University Hospitals Trust. However this came only after a costly[63] and protracted tendering process which consumed large amounts of NHS management time, and after the local community health services trust, (Cambridgeshire Community Services, CCS) had been twice rebuffed in its attempt to win the contract. CCS now has to make hundreds of staff redundant, while the successful NHS bidders are faced with a complex and confusing contract which offered so little prospect of profit that several shortlisted private consortia pulled out before the decision was made.

Nevertheless the Cambridgeshire decision was an important reminder that putting services out to tender does not have to mean that they are privatised. Indeed, while most contracts since the Health and Social Care Act have gone to private bids, a stock-take shows that despite years of erosion and contracting-out since New Labour first devised its Concordat with private hospitals and the Independent Sector Treatment Centres, the majority of NHS-funded care is still delivered by NHS providers and NHS foundation trusts.

A Department of Health spokesman said in September 2014: 'Use of the private sector in the NHS represents only 6 per cent of the total NHS budget – an increase of just 1 per cent since May 2010.'[64]

6 per cent of the English NHS budget is £6.3bn.* This is more significant than it appears because much of the budget for patient care consists of services that the private sector

---

* The higher figure of £10bn, which has been widely cited in the news media based on Department of Health Accounts, is not strictly comparable, since it includes ALL non-NHS spending, including the costs of hiring agency staff to fill vacancies, and services provided by local government.

does not (and does not wish to) provide, so privatisation is concentrated in a few areas of health care.

The Institute for Fiscal Studies concluded from its analysis of figures up to 2012 that: 'Despite large growth in the role of private providers in the delivery of some procedures, the vast majority of care is still provided by NHS hospitals.'[65]

The private sector is interested in elective care, community health services and mental health, so the £6.3bn needs to be seen as a share not of the *total* spend, but as a proportion of the *relevant* spending in the NHS. That is equivalent to 13.2 per cent of the £48bn of the NHS budget for primary care, mental health, community and elective services. Even here, the remaining, crucial 86.8 per cent is still in the public sector – including virtually all of the other clinical services, and 100 per cent of the costly, complex and emergency caseload. There is still plenty of NHS left for us to defend.

Pre-election sensitivity

The long run up to the 2015 election has already begun to put the brakes on some plans to put services out to tender and has made it much harder for ministers to press through highly controversial plans for reconfiguration, cuts and closures in acute hospital services. Regardless of efforts to persuade them otherwise, local communities affected by these schemes have proved utterly resistant to arguments seeking to win their acceptance or acquiescence, putting local MPs of all main parties on the spot if they wish to be re-elected. Panicked by the impending crisis, Jeremy Hunt has suddenly released hundreds of millions of pounds of extra funding to prop up flagging A&E services over the winter in the hopes of minimising angry headlines which may stick in voters' minds as polling day approaches.

In October and November 2014 the government faced the first national action by trade unions on NHS pay since 1982 – further evidence of the unstable political footing of the coalition in its plans for a decade of austerity, cuts and privatisation in the NHS. This included the first-ever strike action by the Royal College of Midwives. Even the proportion of the one million NHS workforce who were not on strike, and those who have meekly put up with the hefty cuts in real terms pay since 2009, are unlikely to warm to parties that insist their pay and conditions have to be sacrificed indefinitely in order to balance the books.

Shortly after his arrival in office Simon Stevens, the NHS England Chief Executive (a man fresh from a decade near the top of the giant US private medical giant UnitedHealth) published the *Five Year Forward View*.[66] It effectively declared its intention to undermine key elements of the Health and Social Care Act, making no reference at all to competition and setting out new proposals to integrate services that have been pushed apart by the Act. Stevens also put the question of NHS finances firmly on the table, demanding an additional 1.5 per cent per year (£8bn) above inflation for the five years from 2015, to come alongside a hugely optimistic, unprecedented £22bn which he hopes to generate through 'efficiency savings'.

All the mainstream parties hurried to declare their support for the Stevens plan and claim some ownership of it. It remains to be seen whether any of them is prepared to agree the additional level of funding he is asking for, or whether any extra money that is planned will be provided soon enough to prevent an escalating crisis from 2015 onwards.

In the run-up to May 2015 and the months to follow, it's all to play for. We have an NHS to win back – or lose. Which will it be?

The Myths About the NHS

For 20 years successive governments have pursued a policy [for the NHS] that the public hasn't voted for and doesn't want.

The Plot against the NHS, Colin Leys and Stewart Player

For two decades politicians have introduced policies for the NHS that ran against the wishes of the vast majority of voters. These policies have been packaged up and sold to us as necessary 'reforms', a useful word suggesting improvements, although this has rarely been the case. They have justified their 'reforms' by a variety of myths about the NHS, which have become received wisdom for many people, including the media, and which are often no longer even questioned.

Before the 2010 election David Cameron promised no more top down reorganisations of the NHS and yet after the election his health secretary, Andrew Lansley, revealed to a bemused public the mother of all reorganisations, so big it could 'be seen from space'. More myths were called for, explaining why the Health and Social Care Bill was necessary at a time when the NHS was rapidly improving with its highest popularity ratings ever. The HSC Act would give power and money to GPs to make the right decisions for their patients, patients would have more choice, the Act would reduce stifling NHS bureaucracy and red tape and would save money in the process. Choice would be improved and efficiency guaranteed by outsourcing NHS care to the carefully named 'independent sector' but this absolutely did not mean that the service was being privatised. The biggest myth has been that the NHS is expensive and inefficient leading to the useful and inevitable conclusion that 'it can't go on like this'.

All these myths have proved to be false, but they have been repeated so often that they are still masquerading as incontrovertible truth even as the evidence accumulates that they are manifestly untrue. This part of the book takes the myths one by one and exposes them for what they are – convenient lies to conceal the continued attempts by an alliance of politicians and commercial interests to dismantle the NHS as a publicly funded, publicly provided and publicly accountable service.

Each of the chapters dealing with a myth is preceded by a short introduction and a summary of the case against for those who might be unfamiliar with the arguments.

2

Myth: The NHS is inefficient and unaffordable. It can't go on like this.

*We cannot afford not to reform the NHS. All I care about is that we avert the crisis and give the NHS the support it needs for the future.** Andrew Lansley

The NHS wasn't broke and it didn't need fixing. John Lister

When the coalition came to power in 2010 the NHS was doing well. Waiting times were falling and outcomes improving, and the service was at its most popular with the public since surveys began. International studies confirmed it as a very cost efficient, equitable and effective service.

Andrew Lansley and David Cameron cherry-picked statistics about clinical outcomes in order to misrepresent it as a failing service, which allowed them to justify their massive and disruptive reforms.

The coalition and their supporters, including right-wing think tanks, also claimed that reform was needed because the NHS was unaffordable.

Although the NHS has been shown to be highly cost effective there is significant wastage, but this is in areas to which politicians and think tanks are deliberately blind. The NHS market in England, set up by Labour and enthusiastically pursued by the Tories, wastes billions of pounds a year but

* http://www.theguardian.com/society/2012/mar/13/nhs-collapse-without-reforms-lansley.

brings no benefits for patients. On the contrary it replaces collaboration with competition, fragments the patient pathway and diverts scarce financial and clinical resources away from frontline activities. At a time of financial pressure it is an ideological indulgence, but no major political party is proposing to fully abandon it.

The NHS needs to concentrate on improving clinical outcomes and patient experience but it needs stability and adequate finances to achieve this. The Health and Social Care Act gave it neither but has rather plunged it into organisational chaos and financial instability. Longer waiting times, rationed treatment and demoralised staff mean that it is the patients who are paying the price.

* * *

Lies, damned lies and statistics

Successive governments have lied repeatedly about the NHS and their lies have taken many forms. They have lied by omitting important facts, they have buried them deep in documents that most people won't read or they have published them when they thought no one was listening ('a good day to bury bad news'). Increasingly they hide inconvenient facts behind 'commercial confidentiality' or they have just stopped gathering data all together so that they can claim with justification that they don't have the facts. Then there is spin. When confronted with other people's facts that need to be denied the political spin machine goes into overdrive and civil servants, whose traditional role was to provide reliable information, are now expected to defend indefensible government policy on the NHS. Finally, when lies and damned lies fail, you can always follow Mark Twain's advice and resort to statistics.

Big lies were called for when the Tories arrived in government and announced their grand top down reorganisation of the NHS. When the Labour government left power in 2010 patient satisfaction levels were the highest since surveys began. Waiting times for inpatients and outpatients had fallen and outcomes were rapidly improving after more money had been put into the NHS for front line care. As John Lister has succinctly pointed out – the NHS wasn't broke and it didn't need fixing.

Andrew Lansley therefore had to justify his expensive disruption of the service and in his efforts to do so the first casualty was truth. He shamelessly cherry-picked statistics to prove that the country's health outcomes were among the poorest in Europe. The media uncritically regurgitated his accusations and obliged him with banner headlines that the UK rate of heart attacks was double that in France and that cancer outcomes were abysmal. The public was suitably alarmed and softened up for the next step, his massive Health and Social Care Bill.

Eventually academics pointed out that Lansley had taken liberties with statistics in order to paint the NHS as a failing service that needed to be rescued by his 'reforms'. John Appleby, chief economist at the King's Fund, wrote an article in the *BMJ*[1] which questioned Lansley's assertions. He demolished the data on heart attack rates, pointing out that not only was the rate falling faster in the UK than in any other European country but had been achieved with less money, with France spending 29 per cent more on health care than the UK. He also showed that the cancer survival data had been cherry-picked and that far from the UK being the 'sick man of Europe' there had been significant improvements in survival rates, with the UK set to have lower death rates than France within a short time. But few members of the public read the *BMJ* and Lansley's purpose had been achieved – voters believed the NHS was failing them and his reforms were needed to rescue it.

We can't go on like this – There is No Alternative

Along with the specific lies about outcomes, the coalition has waged a more general campaign against the NHS. They declared the service to be 'unsustainable', which naturally led to the conclusion that 'we can't carry on like this' and the TINA defence of Lansley's proposed reforms – There is No Alternative. Having frightened the public with dire tales of poor outcomes the politicians didn't really need to be more specific or evidence-based and if they did they cited the cost of the NHS. It was too expensive and inefficient and in times of austerity we couldn't continue to lavish so much money on a failing health service.

But a major international survey showed them to be liars about this too. The Commonwealth Fund is a private US foundation that reports on health systems, using its own data as well as that from other international organisations.[2] Its 2010 report, involving 20,000 patients in 11 developed nations, found that the NHS was one of the most cost-effective healthcare systems with excellent access to care. Only New Zealand, where 1 in 7 had missed out on care because of costs, was cheaper and only Switzerland, spending 35 per cent more, gave better access. Despite the fact that these findings were widely known – and it would have been highly negligent for the Department of Health not to know about them – the government pursued their policy of lying about and denigrating the NHS.

In 2014 the Commonwealth Fund reported again, with an even better result for the NHS. This time it was ranked highest overall, using as criteria quality of care, access to care, efficiency, equity and healthy lives. Bottom of the list on almost all counts was the US system, managing to spend twice as much as other countries while getting worse outcomes and much worse access.[3] Politicians like Hunt were quick to claim credit for the Fund's findings this time, although the success of the NHS was certainly achieved in spite of rather than because of their political interference.

Just as impressive as the top ranking was the fact that the NHS had achieved this while relatively under resourced. In the same year a report from the Office for National Statistics showed that the UK spent the least of the G7 countries (9.2 per cent of GDP) on health care, tying equal bottom with Italy.[4] An EU study reported that the UK was ranked 24th out of 27 EU nations for doctors per capita, worse than Bulgaria and Estonia.[5] An OECD study showed that Britain had fewer hospital beds per person than almost any country in the western world (the second lowest of 23 European countries).[6] It was clear that the NHS was under resourced but still managing to achieve good results in a very cost-effective manner. The vested interests were not deterred and went on claiming that it was unsustainable and unaffordable, and the public began to believe them. Many in the media, led by the *Daily Mail*, were content to keep repeating government lies in their headlines, scaring patients and undermining NHS staff, who were trying to keep the service going under the relentless barrage of criticism.

Lying about NHS finances

In 2010 Cameron had appeared on pre-election posters promising that he would cut the deficit not the NHS, but this turned out to be another lie. The coalition government has subjected the NHS to financial hardship, described by its new CEO Simon Stevens as 'the longest squeeze on NHS finances in our 65 year history'.[7] They have presided over an unprecedented slowdown in the growth of NHS funding, reversing the progress that had been made under the previous government. The so called 'Nicholson challenge'[8] combined with other financial pressures such as PFI contracts are precipitating daily crises for patients and staff as waiting lists rise, treatment is rationed and A&E targets are missed.

A report by the King's Fund in May 2014 warned that a financial crisis was now inevitable and that urgent action was needed to plug the funding gap. Increased spending on the NHS between 1997 and 2010 had pushed the NHS budget up from 5.2 per cent to 8 per cent of GDP but the King's Fund warned that this was heading back down again to 6 per cent by 2021 if nothing changed.[9] The Nuffield Trust followed suit a couple of months later, noting that it was becoming more and more difficult to find further 'efficiency savings', many of which had been at the expense of staff pay freezes and management cuts. They pointed out that the sums involved were not large – the overall trust deficit was just £100m for 2013-14. They also might have mentioned that while frontline care was clearly suffering under the financial squeeze the Treasury had clawed back a £2.2bn 'underspend' from the NHS in 2013, and £1.4bn the previous year.[10] It was notable that the government was quite prepared to see patients suffer while NHS money was returned to the treasury, and that while able to bail out bankers to the tune of billions the government chose not to do the same for the NHS for relatively trivial sums. It began to look to campaigners as though the government was deliberately running down the NHS, calling to mind Chomsky's observation about how to privatise a public service: 'That's the standard technique of privatisation: defund, make sure things don't work, people get angry, you hand it over to private capital.'[11]

Survival of the richest – up-front patient fees

There were many prepared to propose solutions to the NHS financial crisis. Simon Stevens, new CEO of NHS England, deplored the state of NHS finances in his NHS *Five Year Forward Review* and talked about saving money through the usual buzzword bingo of modernisation, embracing new models of care, and shifting work out of hospitals. Think-tanks, some captured by corporate interests, were ready with answers that typically involved up-front patient charges, which would require a radical overthrow of one of the founding principles of the NHS.

The think tank Reform was keen to recommend charges for NHS services ranging from GP visits to 'hotel charges' for hospital inpatients.[12] Lord Warner, a member of the Advisory Council of Reform, co-wrote a *Guardian* article backing Reform's recommendations, in which he attacked the NHS as unaffordable and 'often poor value for money' (having presumably failed to read the Commonwealth Fund report). The solution according to Warner (among other equally unsavoury non-evidence-backed recommendations) was a £10 per month NHS membership scheme.[13] Apparently it hadn't occurred to him that while £120 per year was a trivial sum for a peer (rather less than half the £300 daily attendance rate at the House of Lords) it might well look like an unaffordable amount to many on low (or no) income relying on the NHS for their care.

There are many reasons why patient fees and up front charges are a bad idea. They discourage those who most need the system from using it, meaning delayed presentation and possible worse outcomes. Fees are expensive to means test and collect.

In the US chasing fees costs a fifth of total turnover. In Germany a proposal to collect a fee for GP appointments was abandoned when it was discovered that not only was the cost of means testing and then collecting it prohibitive but that patients on low wages didn't attend their GP as soon as they should have done, and were more likely eventually to need emergency and/or more complex treatment.

See: Kahn JG, Kronick R, Kreger M, Gans DN, 'The cost of health insurance administration in California: estimates for insurers, physicians, and hospitals' in *Health Affairs* (Millwood) 2005;24:1629-39.

Fees for treatment fundamentally alter the doctor-patient relationship – threatening to destroy the trust between doctor and patient – and when patients pay up front they may expect to be treated as customers and sold what they want. Up front charges breach one of the founding principles of the NHS, that care is free at the point of need. Once the principle is breached further charges and top up insurance will follow (it is doubtful whether even Lord Warner believed that his NHS membership fee would remain at £10 per month for very long).

The introduction of fees is a zombie idea – a policy which refuses to die despite being killed by evidence – which is kept alive by right-wing politicians and think tanks. They don't really believe that fees will rescue NHS finances but they do believe that if they can break the principle of free (at the point of need) and equitable NHS treatment then the door to top-up insurance, co-payments and the whole apparatus of a full market in healthcare will open up to them. For these reasons most doctors are vigorously opposed to user charges and upfront fees and maverick motions proposing fees are thrown out at every medical conference.[14]

How to save the NHS money – just get rid of the market

What was noteworthy in the ponderous reports on how to rescue NHS finances was what they didn't mention – the dog that didn't bark in the night. None of them, including Simon Steven's recent review, bothered to address one of the biggest wastages of the English NHS budget, the NHS market.

Since Thatcher introduced an NHS market – the so-called purchaser/provider split – NHS administration costs have escalated. Successive governments have been coy about what they amount to but the generally accepted figures are that pre-market they were 6 per cent, then rose to 12 per cent under Thatcher's internal market, and are now in the region of 15 per cent (in the US the administration costs involved in running health care as a market are estimated to be nudging on 30 per cent). Even by conservative estimates getting rid of the market would save between £5bn and £10bn a year for the English NHS.[15]

The NHS market has done nothing to improve patient care and indeed in 2010 the Commons' Health Select Committee declared it to be a costly failure.[16] Tendering, billing, accounting, chasing fees, legal costs all use up the precious NHS budget and divert money away from frontline care, and these costs have only been exacerbated by the Health and Social Care Act. For instance in 2012 the Audit Commission warned that classifying patients for accounting purposes was wasting valuable NHS time and money which would be better spent on the patients themselves.[17] In 2013 the deputy chair of Monitor complained that the new competition arrangements were 'a bonanza for lawyers and [management] consultants' and could lead to scandals. He made his remarks ahead of a proposed[18] merger of two hospitals which was supported by local doctors but opposed by an unidentified local private hospital. The merger, called for by the NHS hospitals themselves 'to ensure the sustainability of services', was eventually blocked by the Competition Commission on the grounds that it would reduce 'patient choice'.[19] David Lock QC, an expert in NHS contract issues, told the *BMJ*: 'This shows the conflict between running the NHS as a public service and running it as a regulated market.'[20] The lengthy battle over the merger is estimated to have cost the NHS (and thus the taxpayer) almost £2m in consultancy and legal fees.[21]

Competition, prioritised over co-operation in a market-driven NHS, has not been shown to improve patient care. Even the then CEO of NHS England, David Nicholson, complained that the new laws promoting competition were hampering efforts to improve services, citing the blocked merger of the two trusts, and examples of GP practices not being allowed to federate.[22] But, despite the lack of evidence, Lansley placed competition at the heart of the Health and Social Care Act and section 75, the HSCA regulations on competition, represented yet another Lansley lie. He had originally promised GPs that 'it was absolutely not the case' that Clinical Commissioning Groups (CCGs) would have to put services out to tender, and Earl Howe had promised those concerned about the regulations that there would be 'no legal obligation to create new markets'. But the legislation showed them to be liars yet again.

After the passage of the infamous section 75 legislation Professor Martin McKee, in an article in the *BMJ*, lamented that the NHS was now at the mercy of lawyers, including some of the peers who had supported the Act

The future of healthcare in England lies in the hands not of politicians and professionals but of competition lawyers. Clinical commissioning groups … will think twice before invoking the wrath of one of the large corporations now moving into healthcare. With legal and contracting teams many times larger than those available to the commissioners, it is they who will be the ultimate arbiters of the shape of healthcare.[23]

There have already been expensive challenges from the private sector over the awarding of contracts and anecdotal reports of CCGs allowing contracts to remain with private firms[24] because of the fear of the legal costs of not doing so.

Despite the expense and the perverse consequences there seems to be no political will to abandon the English NHS market and use the billions that would be freed up for patient care instead.[25] But of course having an NHS market in place is necessary to enable the privatisation of the English NHS, another policy which is wasting money hand over fist with no benefit for patients (see Chapter 8).

Improving NHS finances

There are other ways of improving the NHS finances. PFI projects are crippling many hospitals and the debate is now raging about how to reclaim hospitals and the eye watering PFI repayments (which put Wonga in the shade) from the hands of the rapacious private sector. Significant amounts of money are being wasted on agency staff. Trusts were panicked and sacked permanent staff to save money – but then were forced to fill the gaps with agency staff after the Francis report called for safe staffing levels. The Nuffield Trust estimated that foundation trust spending on agency staff had risen by 27 per cent (£300m) in 2013-14, wiping out any savings from the sackings.[26] Unfortunately short term thinking and the exigencies of the Health and Social Care Act – demanding competition at the expense of collaboration – mean that many ways of saving money are for the moment out of bounds.

There is of course a wider debate to be had when it comes to NHS funding. Would patients rather have Trident or treatment (unfortunately the government is not offering that particular patient choice)? Why not a hypothecated tax[27] or Robin Hood tax for the NHS, or just make sure that corporate taxes are paid – dealing with tax avoidance (£25bn a year) and tax evasion (£70bn a year) would produce more than enough money to bail out the NHS and put it on a stable footing. The politicians have answers to their manufactured and avoidable NHS funding crisis but are not prepared to use them.

Conclusion

The current crisis in the English NHS is largely down to repeated politically imposed 're-disorganisations' and to arbitrary financial pressures. Failed political initiatives are followed not by insight or apologies but calls for yet more change because previous changes didn't work. Against this background of government incompetence politicians and establishment NHS watchers complain that the NHS is unsustainable and unaffordable but the NHS market in England – a very costly failure – is still in place for what can only be ideological reasons. No major political party shows any inclination to fully remove the market despite all the evidence against it. No major health think tank seems able to grasp the nettle and recommend that it is abolished.

Expensive PFI projects, forced on trusts as 'the only game in town', are now causing trusts to fail – triggering cuts in other local hospitals and services. Privatisation has resulted in more money being wasted – staff time and resources are being squandered through compulsory tendering, and the NHS budget is going to shareholders and tax havens instead of frontline care. Enforced competition means NHS institutions can no longer collaborate to help patients. Staff have seen real earnings fall and work under the constant threat of their services being outsourced, cut or closed. Insecurity, criticism and fear do not produce a work place that is conducive to good patient care, but this is what staff face every day.

The English NHS isn't perfect and campaigners have never

pretended otherwise, but in order to improve and remain patient-centred it needs stability and adequate funding and it has neither at the moment. The miracle is that despite political incompetence and meddling NHS staff still manage to deliver a good service to patients in what looks increasingly like a war zone.

The NHS has proved itself over the years to be a good model for delivering health care. It is cost effective, equitable and after appropriate investment was achieving good outcomes for patients with whom it is extremely popular. For 65 years it has allowed us to live free of the fear of the financial consequences of illness. Repeated assertions that it is unsustainable and unaffordable have no foundation, and should be challenged whenever they appear. And those who maintain that we cannot afford the NHS must be made to answer the most important question – if we can't afford the most cost-effective health service in the world what can we afford?

3

Myth: Our NHS reforms will mean more choice for patients.

Cameron said that greater competition within the NHS was the key to enhanced patient choice.

The Daily Telegraph, 20 August 2009[1]

The Health and Social Care Act 2012 requires commissioners to ensure good practice and to promote and protect patient choice.

NHS England document 'Choice and Competition'[2]

Patient choice is integral to patient dignity and respect and lies at the heart of the doctor-patient relationship. It is very difficult to argue against. Politicians have exploited that fact to produce their own version of patient choice, which serves their ideological direction for the NHS rather than the patient. They have maintained that choice requires an increased number of providers of NHS care, which has in turn been the reason for opening the NHS up to the private sector, creating an NHS market in England.

The Health and Social Care Act has facilitated competition and marketisation of the NHS, always in the name of patient choice. But patients and their doctors have less choice now than they did when the NHS was first founded. The choices that most patients want – a good local hospital, a familiar GP who has the ability to refer them for specialist care when necessary – are increasingly under threat because of

Lansley's 'reforms'. CCGs are bound by contracts, referral management centres may deny the choices that doctors and their patients make and the awarding of profitable work to the private sector threatens to undermine local NHS services which the private sector can't and won't provide.

True patient choice does not require the NHS to compete with the private sector nor does it need a full blown NHS market. Indeed as the private sector takes over the delivery of more NHS care it is they who will pick and choose which patients they will take on. Patient choice is important but only when it is meaningful to patients, not when it is a means of facilitating a political agenda.

* * *

True choice versus politically driven patient choice

Before the NHS was founded in 1948, choice for patients was limited. Individuals were able to choose their GP, dentist and optician, but choice did not extend any further. Many had no choice at all, denied access to health care by their poverty. With the advent of the NHS previously unaffordable services became available to everyone, and people rushed to sign up, forcing many initially reluctant GPs to join the NHS that they and the BMA had originally opposed.

GPs, even those who had been most sceptical about the new NHS, were able to refer any of their patients for any treatment they required, and to prescribe drugs in the knowledge that price would no longer prevent poorer patients receiving them. Hospital doctors were enabled for the first time to link up at local level with colleagues in what had previously been other small, rival hospitals, to share knowledge, collaborate in the development of new services, and treat a much wider cross-section of people.[3] As a result, from 1948 until 1991 (which saw the creation of the NHS internal market) patient choice was a reality, a genuine entity, and included the possibility that health authorities could purchase care in the private sector if they so wished.

While the patient choice on offer during that period may have been sufficient for health professionals and their patients it was not the sort of choice that served the purposes of right-wing politicians and the private sector. Above all it did not allow private companies to get a foot in the door of the NHS and their hands on its guaranteed budget. That required the creation of a market. Markets mean competition and competition requires an increased number of providers alongside the NHS. Who better to step in and fill the gap than the private sector? The competition thus created would result in better outcomes for patients by driving up standards and would give patients the holy grail of health care, more 'patient choice'. Or so the argument went.

Thus began the process of marketising the NHS, for which political intervention was required. As Paul Corrigan (Alan Milburn's health advisor) remarked[4] – The state has to actively create a market, they don't appear of their own account. Politicians always justified the policies required as a drive for more patient choice, to be achieved through increased competition. The public was introduced to a lexicon of weasel words to explain the changes. Competition was downgraded to 'contestability', while the scrum of private companies descending on the NHS was reassuringly described as 'a plurality of providers'. 'World class commissioning' would make the NHS more 'patient-centred'. The process was misrepresented, concealed behind a screen of vaguely comforting but meaningless jargon, all intended to divert the public from what was really going on – politicians were turning the NHS into a market, with health as its commodity, and open to the private sector who were after their holy grail, the guaranteed funds of the NHS budget.

It is not surprising therefore that patient choice, ostensibly as wholesome and desirable as motherhood and apple pie, began to be viewed with distrust by many who understood how the concept was being abused to justify the creation of an NHS market. 'Patient choice' has been used by successive governments as the Trojan horse to facilitate the introduction of the private sector into the NHS, and ironically the more politicians have championed it the less of it there has been.

A short history of competition in the NHS

The HSC Act has opened the door to a full-blooded market in the English NHS but the story of competition and establishing a market goes much further back.

The covert conversion of the NHS into a business started with the Griffiths report in 1983 (see separate box). Then in January 1988 (in the midst of a serious 'winter crisis' triggered by spending cuts in the aftermath of the 1987 general election) Margaret Thatcher used an interview on television to announce that she was going to conduct a 'review' of the NHS. There was widespread trepidation, since her major confrontation with the miners in 1984 had been preceded by a 'review' of the coal industry. Her NHS review was even more secretive and exclusive and only a small circle of chosen Thatcher supporters was involved. Just over 12 months later on 31 January 1989 Margaret Thatcher made a speech announcing the outcome of the review: a new NHS White Paper 'Working for Patients'.[5] In it she said: 'We aim to extend patient choice, to delegate responsibility to where the services are provided.'

Griffiths Report

In 1983, at the height of the Thatcher administration, Roy Griffiths (a director and deputy chair of the Sainsbury's supermarket chain from 1968-1991), was asked to write a report on NHS management. The Griffiths Report consisted of just 24 pages of assertions without any supporting evidence and called for a major change: Griffiths recommended that the Secretary of State should set up, within the Department of Health and Social Security and the existing statutory framework, a Health Services Supervisory Board and a full-time NHS Management Board

At local level, general managers should be introduced throughout the NHS.

This was a move away from the old management structure and began the process of replacing administrators who were steeped in the values of the NHS with managers who might be drawn from outside the NHS, including the private sector. This in effect started the NHS down a path of seeing itself as a business.[6] Interestingly the 1983 Griffiths Report also called for GPs to get more involved in budgets and commissioning of services – a trend that culminated in Lansley's White Paper of 2010.

For his 'services to the NHS' Griffiths was rewarded with a knighthood in 1985.

So began the 25-year non-evidence-based experiment which has attempted to turn the NHS into a market-based system, and the emphasis on choice as a justification for these market-based reforms has been a constant theme of politicians ever since. Thatcher went on to say: 'All of the proposals in this White Paper put the needs of patients first … the patient's needs will always be paramount.'

Thatcher's reforms were pushed through Parliament in 1990 (despite very substantial opposition, including a major advertising campaign by the BMA) as the National Health Service and Community Care Act. This created a new 'internal market' in the NHS by dividing up the previously integrated District Health Authorities and by separating off hospitals, mental health and other services, which were expected to 'opt out' of direct NHS control and become NHS trusts. The Health Authorities themselves were to be set up as 'purchasers', and given the budget to buy services from 'providers' on behalf of their local population. Another aspect of the reforms was to give GPs (who then became 'GP fundholders') their own budgets to purchase services for their own patients. This handed budgets directly to larger GP practices to allow them to go out to the marketplace and buy services such as blood testing or knee replacements. The whole effect was to introduce the 'purchaser provider split', essentially a primitive market in which health authorities and some GPs held the budgets to purchase care from 'providers'. At this stage the market – for all its divisiveness and extra overhead costs – was 'internal' to the NHS, and virtually none of the money for clinical care was being diverted to the private sector.

John Major's government published The Patients' Charter in 1991 (revised in 1995). This affirmed the right of every citizen to be referred to a consultant, acceptable to the patient, when the patient's GP felt it necessary. Although the Charter was seen as weak overall, it helped to establish the importance of putting patients at the centre of care.

Choice was not an immediate priority for the new Labour Government when it came to power in its landslide win in 1997. However in 2000 Alan Milburn, as Health Secretary, signed a 'Concordat' with private hospitals under which the NHS would pay (up to 40 per cent above the NHS cost) for the treatment in private wards of waiting list patients whose operations had been delayed due to winter pressures. This was a 'choice' to be made by the NHS rather than the patient.[7] It was not until 2002 that plans were announced to offer patients who were already on waiting lists opportunities to choose alternative providers. Milburn was again the chief architect of this, advised by Simon Stevens, now the Chief Executive of NHS England.

It was at this time that 'patient choice' began to be referred to as a policy objective in its own right. At the same time, the government changed the system of hospital payment, to support the policy of patient choice. Payment by Results (PbR)* introduced a fixed tariff payment per case treated and was a further mechanism for diverting NHS money to the private sector.

Payment by Results

PbR was, in theory, supposed to be a way of creating strong incentives for hospitals to raise income by attracting and treating more patients. However it was also a way to ensure that any patients who 'chose' or were induced to seek treatment from a private provider took the money with them out of the NHS. This made possible the division of what had previously been 'block contracts' between purchasers and provider trusts, often covering the whole local population. In this way PbR deliberately destabilised NHS trusts, leaving them uncertain how many patients they would treat and therefore how much money they could expect to receive to pay staff and suppliers

By contrast the contracts for Labour's new invention, 'Independent Sector Treatment Centres', purpose-built small scale private units, owned and run by mainly overseas for-profit providers, were unbelievably generous. The ISTCs were given five-year contracts, far longer than any NHS hospitals could hope for, and guaranteed numbers of patients, regardless of how few chose to use the new units, with a special tariff price averaging 11 per cent above the

---

* Interestingly nothing to do with results (outcomes) of treatment in terms of the health of the patient, which is not taken into account; it is simply a fixed tariff of payments for each treatment, based on the average costs of NHS providers.

going NHS rate for each job.

The Blair government, egged on by Milburn, Stevens and others, was artificially creating a new market in health care by preferentially favouring these new for-profit providers. NHS trusts were even forbidden from bidding for the ISTC contracts, and negotiations on many of the deals were taken out of the hands of local purchasers and conducted at national level by Department of Health bureaucrats. When members of one local Primary Care Trust objected to a deal being done on their behalf and without consultation, the objecting board members were abruptly removed.

By the time the Labour Government lost power in 2010, the concept of patient choice in the NHS was firmly established. In May 2010 the coalition government launched their white paper 'Liberating the NHS' in which competition and choice were inextricably linked. Choice lay at the heart of the proposals but could only be had through competition. Competition in turn required a plurality of 'Any Willing Providers' which meant an expanding role for the private sector. The market had won out in a one-sided argument, and choice was its sharpest weapon.

Any Willing Provider

The Health and Social Care Bill introduced the concept of 'Any Willing Provider', which allows private companies and other non-NHS bodies to bid for lucrative NHS contracts. In theory to qualify they must satisfy a bureaucratic and cumbersome process, which is a burden for any small charity or third sector organisation to navigate but suits large multinational organisations perfectly. The term 'Any Willing Provider' was quietly changed with no fanfare to 'Any Qualified Provider' (AQP) to try and make the process sound more professional and less like a free for all in the NHS contract bidding process.

Many CCG websites explain to the public that AQP is 'a work programme that will enable the Government to fulfil its commitment to *increase choice and personalisation* in NHS funded services for patients and the public'. Andrew Lansley himself, speaking to a 2011 conference of GPs said: 'Of course, patient choice implies competition ... there are areas where there is already strong demand for more choice – such as community services. This is where we will begin to introduce any qualified provider.'

The Department of Health lists the strategic aims of AQP as to:

- Increase choice and access of health service providers for patients.
- Improve quality and outcomes of health services.
- Drive innovation and efficiency of health service.

Most campaigners, remembering the multitude of new, low quality cleaning and other companies which set up to cash in when the Thatcher government opened up hospital cleaning and other ancillary services to competitive tendering back in the mid-1980s see AQP as a tool to allow profit-seeking companies large or small to take over NHS services.

What has really happened to patient choice?

Patient choice should of course be at the heart of health care but it must be the choice that patients really want, not a spurious version that only serves the aims of the private sector. Most patients for instance want a good quality, local and responsive NHS available to treat them for their general ailments when necessary. Many patients accept they will have to travel further afield for very specialised care but the principle of a high quality district general hospital close to home is one cherished by most people in the UK. It is deliverable by the NHS, and affordable despite all the protestations of politicians and captured think tanks. Perversely the fragmentation and privatisation of the NHS resulting from the HSC Act, along with cuts and closures, threaten this most basic of patient choices. All over the country groups of campaigners are organising to protect local services and struggling to make themselves heard[8] – a travesty of Lansley's promise that there would be no decision about you without you, and a denial of patient choice on a grand scale.

At the same time the genuine patient choice that existed in the first decades of the NHS has been eroded by the very mechanisms that were recently introduced allegedly to promote it. Originally GPs could refer patients anywhere and to any other doctor working in the NHS. With the introduction of the market such referrals are increasingly tied to the contracts that CCGs enter into, with special arrangements required for patients who wish to be seen elsewhere. The following illustration appeared in the comment columns of the *Guardian* in November 2013:

Following a disastrous A&E experience at Hinchingbrooke Hospital (and our closest A&E at Kettering being under a 'black notice' due to staff shortages), we ended up at Bury St Edmunds A&E who diagnosed my partner as requiring surgery on her knee. We arranged through the consultant at Bury for the surgery to be carried out at Addenbrookes by a surgeon who had already performed similar surgery on my partner's son with spectacular success.

All well and good until we were summoned by a GP at a [Northamptonshire] Practice ... where we were told in no uncertain terms that the operation would be carried out by a surgeon at Milton Keynes who is not even a specialist in this area.

The reason given – 'this is who my contract is with'. When we then questioned what would happen if we went to Addenbrookes anyway, we were told we would have to fund the surgery ourselves. He delivered this information with a poster headed 'NHS Choices' taped to the wall behind him.[9]

Patient choice is also seriously threatened by CCGs' use of referral management centres, designed to reduce the number – and thus the cost to CCGs – of patients being referred to hospital for specialist opinion. Referral letters, written to specialists by GPs who know and will have examined their patients, may be redirected to less specialised services, queried and thus delayed or simply declined by staff who may have little or no clinical experience. This not only makes a mockery of the promise of more patient choice but is clinically dangerous, with examples of delays to patients needing urgent specialist opinion and treatment. At the same time Jeremy Hunt, in a spectacular failure of joined up thinking, is threatening doctors who 'cost patients' lives by failing to send them for vital hospital tests soon enough'.[10]

True patient choice is further eroded by the threat posed to local services by the private sector. Elsewhere in the book evidence is provided to show how the privatisation of cherry-picked services can easily undermine the local NHS, which is left providing the expensive and emergency services that are of no interest to the private sector.

BBC's *Newsnight* recently[11] produced a short film extolling the private sector delivery of NHS elective surgery because some individuals interviewed rated the private care they received slightly more highly than NHS care. But if those same patients understood that their local NHS services were threatened by the local private sector contract they might take that into account when assessing the desirability of that contract. The price paid for the choice of an NHS hip replacement in a private hospital may look too high if the consequence is the destabilisation and possible loss of local NHS orthopaedic and trauma services. The private hospital will not be interested in that same patient when they fracture their hip or need complex orthopaedic treatment that the private firm is not contracted to deliver. The argument is far more complex than *Newsnight* suggested and patients and the public deserve a much better account of it from supposedly responsible media.

The tendering out of sexual health services also provides a classic example of how patients may end up with less choice, limited access and a worse service once the private sector takes over a contract. In 2013 representatives of the UK's hospital doctors and sexual health specialists wrote to all local councils in England strongly advising them not to put services that provide contraception and diagnose sexually transmitted infections out to competitive tender.[12] They claimed that outsourcing posed several 'key threats', including reduced access to clinics and treatment and a reduction in the quality of patient care and added:

> Tendering has negatively impacted on the provision of sexual health services, destabilising, disintegrating and fragmenting services, causing significant uncertainty amongst patients and staff, and reducing overall levels of patient care.[13]

Is competition needed for patient choice?

The cost of imposing competition on the English NHS is high both in terms of the money wasted on running a market (upwards of £5bn a year), and in the deleterious affect it has on the service. Other chapters describe the perverse effects for patients of competition rather than collaboration, and the cost and disruption of the plethora of competition lawyers crawling over and profiting from the NHS market. Recently NHS England was forced to concede that there was a 'paucity of evidence' that choice and competition produced any benefit to patients.[14] Their policy director admitted that 'the direct evidence of where best competition and choice works to improve outcomes is fairly limited' – a shocking admission about a policy which has been used to transform the English NHS into a market place and which has wasted untold amounts of NHS money at a time when the service is suffering severe financial pressures.

But, as Professor Calum Paton points out in his review for CHPI, it is perfectly possible to abolish the market and yet still provide patients with choice. GPs can refer patients to an NHS provider of choice, as they once used to. Paton concludes:

Just as markets may not involve choice, choice does not require markets except in the basic sense that plural provision exists. Choice existed from 1948 to 1991, after which the market restricted it. The challenge in the 1980s was to improve the resource allocation formula through regional strategy: then the mechanisms to reconcile choice with effective service reconfiguration would have existed. But this agenda seemed dull to the 1980s Thatcherites who wished to marketise the NHS for ideological reasons. And this dull but valuable truth has been lost over 25 years of exciting but damaging market hegemony.[15]

Since the 1980s, the concept of choice has been used not so much as a way to improve the patient experience but as a lever to replace the planning of services with competition, and a device to carve out a share of NHS budgets to bolster a private sector that has no chance of surviving without extensive government patronage. As Paton shows, competition, so destructive and expensive, was never necessary to provide choice, and indeed as the privatisation of the NHS proceeds choices available to patients will reduce. The private sector is not keen on competition, preferring large monopolies, and patient choice is already on its way to becoming yet another myth. The real choice that patients want – a good reliable local hospital, a familiar GP who knows you and listens – are under significant threat in the new marketised NHS. In future the real choice is likely to lie with those providing health care. They will choose fit, young and profitable patients and reject the elderly, the chronically sick and those with complex problems, as already happens in the US.

London GP Jonathon Tomlinson summed up choice thus on his excellent blog:

Patient choices are integral to dignity and respect and are at the heart of medical ethical principles and the doctor-patient relationship. This is why doctors are so sensitive to criticism that we do not care about patient choice. The reason so many of us who care for patients every day object so strongly to the way that patient choice is framed in the NHS reforms, is that patients and their choices are not being treated as ends in themselves, but merely as means to an end; they are to become subservient to the goals of market based competitive healthcare.[16]

4

Myth: Our NHS reforms will put GPs in the driving seat.

So let's be clear – our aim is a major transfer of responsibility to the GP community; in order to empower clinical decision making and improve outcomes for patients.[1]

Andrew Lansley

You will have the freedom to work with whoever you want to in commissioning health services.[2]

Andrew Lansley

When Andrew Lansley presented the Health and Social Care Bill to a surprised audience he was emphatic that the intention was to hand power and money to GPs. Initially 80 per cent, (subsequently downgraded to 60 per cent) of the NHS budget was to pass to Clinical Commissioning Groups run by GPs who would make the right decisions for their patients, with minimum interference from central government.

The reality has proved to be quite different. Few GPs have the enthusiasm, time or expertise to take on the work involved and the number of GPs on CCGs has declined. Faced with diminishing resources and driven by central diktats CCGs have limited choices and hard decisions to make about how to save money and ration care. Contrary to firm government promises CCGs now have to tender out almost all services, wasting money and clinical time and resulting in an increasing number of contracts going to the private sector.

Some CCG work is already being undertaken by Commissioning Support Units, due to be outsourced in 2016. CCGs are likely to find they have little to do apart from rubber stamp their decisions and those coming down from NHS England, and take the blame for problems. The majority of GPs now believe that they have been set up to take the blame for rationing health care.

Some of the GPs remaining on CCGs have interests in the private health companies bidding for their CCG services, giving rise to conflicts of interest hitherto unknown in the NHS.

* * *

At the heart of Lansley's legislation were two attractive and important promises. One was that patients would be at the centre of the NHS, their choices paramount, a promise encapsulated in the repeated undertaking that there would be 'no decision about you without you'. The other was that GPs would be given the majority of the NHS budget to buy care for patients as they and their patients saw fit. GPs knew best what patients needed and were to be given the power and the money to deliver it. Time and again GPs were told they would be 'in the driving seat', with control of the NHS budget, and that they would be calling the shots on behalf of their patients. These promises have turned out to be worthless, a deliberate deception of GPs and the public.

Lansley's HSC Bill proposed radical structural changes to primary care, with the abolition of 150 Primary Care Trusts as local commissioners of services and the creation of a larger number of new bodies – Clinical Commissioning Groups (CCGs) – to take their place. It was clear from the outset that the proposed changes would have a significant impact on primary care and on the working life of all GPs.

Many opponents of the Bill questioned whether the majority of GPs had the interest, time or expertise to commission services on such a large scale and some also doubted that the government intended to keep their word about handing so much power to GPs. Both doubts were soon justified. GP commissioning turned out to be the bait in the bear trap, used to lure GP leaders who should have known better into accepting legislation which would be disastrous for primary care. As a result GPs have ended up with 'less money, more complexity and all of the blame'.[3] At the same time the HSC Act has opened up key sections of the NHS – including now the work of commissioning – to the private sector, which is increasingly displacing GPs when it comes to making decisions about where and how to spend the NHS budget. Many of the new contracts being offered up for competitive tender focus on a new 'lead provider' which will 'coordinate' services and allocate resources.[4]

Diminishing presence

GPs are supposedly elected to their roles on Clinical Commissioning Groups by their locality GP peers for a period of three years, although many posts are uncontested: in 2011, as the shadow CCGs were formed, research by *Pulse* magazine found 95 per cent of board members had not faced any electoral process.[5] Board members have a say in the policy and commissioning decisions of the CCG, but these GPs can often spend as little as one or two half days per week on CCG business. This leaves much of the real day-to-day work to be undertaken by managers (many re-employed after being made redundant as PCTs closed down) or by Commissioning Support Units, run by NHS England – units which will have to be put out to competitive tender and possible privatisation by 2016. Perhaps one or two GPs in a CCG, such as the clinical chair, will spend three or four days a week on CCG business.

Clinical Commissioning Groups (CCGs)

According to the national body, the NHS Clinical Commissioners (NHSCC),[6] CCGs are:

- Membership bodies, with local GP practices as the members;
- Led by an elected Governing Body made up of GPs, other clinicians including a nurse and a secondary care consultant, and lay members;

- Responsible for about 60 per cent of the NHS budget; or £60 billion per year;
- Responsible for commissioning health care such as mental health services, urgent and emergency care, elective hospital services, and community care;
- Independent, and accountable to the Secretary of State for Health through NHS England;
- Responsible for the health of populations ranging from under 100,000 to 900,000, although the average population covered by a CCG is about a quarter of a million people.

NHSCC also explains that: 'CCGs work closely with NHS England, who have three roles in relation to CCGs. The first is assurance: NHS England has a responsibility to assure themselves that CCGs are fit for purpose, and are improving health outcomes. Secondly, NHS England must help support the development of CCGs. Finally, NHS England are also direct commissioners, responsible for highly specialised services and primary care. As co-commissioners, CCGs work with NHS England's Local Area Teams to ensure joined-up care.'

A survey undertaken by *GP* magazine via a freedom of Information request[7] found that GPs now make up less than half of CCG Board members. Of 2,720 Board members, just 1,188 are GPs. This leaves them in a minority if any votes are taken, so they can hardly be described as being 'in control'.

The FoI request also showed a rapid increase in the number of GPs abandoning their role on CCGs. In one three month period in 2013, 51 GPs gave up their role whilst 68 quit in the whole of 2012. There seems to be a general loss of interest as GPs realise how little influence they really have. CCGs have to follow the diktats from central government and try to make ends meet with budgets that are frozen in real terms whilst demand for health care increases, a far cry from the power and influence they were promised.

A report by the King's Fund[8] showed GPs had limited understanding of the governance arrangements of CCGs and of the constitution that governs them. There was significant disparity of views between those GPs involved in CCGs and those not involved. For example, 81 per cent of CCG leaders felt that decisions made by the CCG reflected their views and those of colleagues, compared with 38 per cent of those without a formal role on the CCG. Many respondents to the survey were highly sceptical of the notion of the CCG being owned by local GPs and saw the CCG as an administrative structure sitting above practices rather than something that is composed of and led by its member GPs.

Rationing care – the blame game

Lansley argued that GPs had wanted more influence for years, and that handing them the budget would allow local control by the very doctors who knew their patients best. But he had also calculated that at a time of increasing financial constraints GP commissioning offered a perfect opportunity for politicians to blame any resulting problems on 'local decision making' and thus absolve themselves of responsibility.* In June 2014 Kailash Chand wrote: 'The NHS bashing, which is now an almost daily feature from politicians needs stopping. Hunt, instead of naming and shaming GPs,

* It is no accident that the very first changes spelled out in Lansley's Bill removed the duty of the Secretary of State to provide comprehensive and universal health services.

please invest in training, education and funding in primary care.'[9] Jeremy Hunt accused GP leaders of scaremongering when concerns were raised about general practice. Mention is made elsewhere of Hunt threatening to name and shame GPs for not referring patients for enough hospital tests while at the same time CCGs are encouraging them to keep patients away from hospitals in order to save money.[10]

Despite reassurances to the contrary from politicians, the coalition has effectively frozen NHS funding since 2010, leading to severe financial pressures on the whole service. Primary care has had to bear more than its share of the burden. Yet the share of NHS budget allocated to primary care has been reduced year by year,[11] while GPs are laden with greater responsibilities and are now increasingly faced with inspection of the work they do.

Funding of GP services is controlled nationally by NHS England and its 'local area teams'. However it is up to CCGs to find ways of saving money by cutting back on services. So far they have largely failed to come up with any proposals that might be acceptable to their local population, while campaigners in many areas are quite rightly watching CCGs like hawks for any sign of cuts that will damage patients. Many of these schemes also have the effect of dumping additional responsibility and work onto primary care and GPs. Often these plans include closing local A&E departments and/or whole hospitals (e.g. in north-west London). But, even then, when they are planning important changes, CCGs often do not bother to consult with local GPs.

One common way in which CCGs are seeking to reduce spending is to cut back on the number of patients that GPs refer to hospitals. Each visit to an outpatient department can cost up to £150 per patient and with investigations charged on top of this, the bill to the CCG soon adds up. Research by the *BMJ* in 2013[12] showed CCGs began implementing restrictions on referrals to secondary care soon after they came into existence in April 2013, at a time when budgets were being squeezed centrally and the so-called 'Nicholson challenge'[13] to generate £20bn savings in the five years to 2015 had to be pursued at all costs.

Sometimes the restrictions on referrals could be defended (such as some for tattoo removal or cosmetic surgery) but it was apparent that in some areas many procedures that might benefit patients were also being rationed or simply made unavailable on the NHS. Ever inventive, CCGs – following the recommendations of the 2009 McKinsey report[14] – attempted to justify rationing by labelling them 'procedures of limited clinical value'. These included procedures such as surgery for Dupuytren's contracture (a disabling hand condition) and for various types of hernia as well as joint replacements. The Royal College of Surgeons[15] argued that dealing with these problems at an early stage would prevent complications later on but the demands of the balance sheet by and large overrode clinical considerations.

Individual GPs are able to appeal to a local panel if they feel their patient should receive treatment that is excluded from their CCG's list of approved procedures. However this can lead to some difficult dilemmas. It is not unknown for a GP, acting on behalf of a patient, to support an appeal against a policy that he or she has signed up to, as a member of a CCG.

If some GPs may ultimately benefit from CCGs 'drawing a line in the sand' when facing difficult decisions about restricting treatments, many others in the profession may be concerned that GPs are being set up to take the blame for rationing care. Either way, the burden was to be borne by the patient denied treatment who was faced then with the choice between going private or going without.

Conflicts of interest

CCGs purchase everything except some specialist care and primary care itself and thus decide where NHS funds are spent in the local health economy. This role seems set to expand, since NHS England is now pressing for CCGs to take over responsibility for 'co-commissioning' primary care,[16] as well as awarding contracts for certain initiatives and services needed in primary care – such as minor surgery services or evening and weekend GP services ('out of hours' services). There has also recently been a move to make them responsible for more of the 'specialist services' such as renal dialysis, although whether the funding will follow is unclear.

They are already responsible for commissioning most acute services – allocating the funds needed to commission a mix of services from the local hospital, for example. These contracts can be sizeable and as we will see many GPs have a financial stake in the companies bidding for them. Conflicts of interest arise when the GPs on commissioning groups might benefit financially from the awarding of such contracts.

This problem was predicted and predictable. Right from the outset, when CCGs were suggested by Lansley, concerns arose over possible conflicts of interest for GPs on CCG governing bodies. It was thought that these could be avoided if any GPs with a direct conflict of interest excused themselves from the discussion when contracts were awarded. This has led to situations where the majority of GPs on a CCG have been unable to vote on awarding a contract, highlighting the ethical dilemmas of 'GP commissioning'. It also raises the question of how reasonable it is to expect decisions to be made without bias when the majority of those responsible for awarding a contract stand to benefit from it financially, even if they have to leave the room for the decision. In Bedfordshire, for example, the CCG awarded a controversial contract for Musculoskeletal (MSK) services to a privately-led consortium including a company owned by almost half the GP practices in Bedfordshire. It got around the problem of brazen conflict of interest by claiming that the decision had been taken by consensus, without a vote.[17] (see Chapter 8)

A conflict of interest occurs, for example, in Blackpool CCG, where five out of the nine GP members of its governing body have an interest in Fylde Coast Medical Services – the private company that runs the GP out of hours (OOH) service,[18] and five have an interest in Virgin Care. Out of hours services are organised and put out to tender by CCGs, so in Blackpool a majority of GPs will have to leave the meeting during any debate or vote on contracts for OOH care. Of the eighteen members on the governing body of this CCG nine are GPs. This doesn't give a majority for the 'GP led organisation' that Lansley championed. In many other CCGs the GPs are in a tiny minority on the governing body, with some running with as few as two or three GPs.

Up against the ramshackle CCG Boards, with part-time GP board members often having varying conflicts of interest, the private sector has organised itself to take best advantage of the situation. Virgin Care Ltd was formed in 2010, marking a re-entry of Richard Branson's company into an NHS market they had previously abandoned. Virgin acquired a majority stake in Assura Medical, which had begun under New Labour as a property company investing in GP premises, but which subsequently moved into primary care.[19] In October

2012, with the HSC Bill six months from implementation, the savvy Virgin Care took over 100 per cent ownership of Assura. But fearing adverse publicity over their joint ventures with GP surgeries, Virgin decided to sever its partnership arrangements and run NHS services themselves.[20] Virgin Care were involved in 343 GP practices running them as 50:50 partnerships; but when the new CCGs were formed 289 GPs divested themselves of their interests, to give them a free hand as commissioners. The last thing Virgin wanted was for local GPs to be criticised in the press, thus making them nervous about the joint work they do with Virgin. Severing the partnerships and establishing sole control of the services gave Virgin a free run to bid for services without needing to worry about conflicts of interest. Virgin continues to run GP surgeries directly as well as many NHS contracts across England. In the usual management speak they justified their decision to ensure 'more consistency of governance and leadership, and efficient use of management resources'.

Virgin Care?

The way in which Virgin maximises profits in primary care by cutting costs, often by employing fewer GPs, was highlighted in 2013 in a feature article in *Red Pepper* magazine, which pointed to the example of the King's Heath practice in Northampton, taken over by Virgin in October 2010. There, three GPs had been reduced to one, and patients found they were waiting three weeks for an appointment rather than the previous three days. At one point the service was delivered by locums for a five month spell while the sole GP was on leave, and the promised 'extended surgery opening hours' meant the premises were open but with no clinical staff present.[21]

Compulsory tendering

During the passage of the HSC Bill Lansley and his colleagues repeatedly reassured GPs that they would be able to choose how to spend the allocated budget. Lansley promised specifically that GPs would not have to put all services out to tender.

> You will ... be able to determine where integrated services are required and commission them accordingly. You will be able to work with existing providers of health and care services to deliver better results for patients. Or you will be able to commission new services to address weaknesses in current levels of provision.
>
> I know many of you may have read that you will be forced to fragment services, or to put services out to tender. This is absolutely not the case. It is a fundamental principle of the Bill that you as commissioners, not the Secretary of State and not regulators, should decide when and how competition should be used to serve your patients' interests. The healthcare regulator, Monitor, would not have the power to force you to put services out to competition.
>
> Andrew Lansley,
> Secretary of State for Health, letter to all GPs,
> 16 February 2012[22]

Of course, we now know that Lansley's promise that GPs would decide whether to tender services has proved to be yet another lie. The promise was brushed aside by the introduction of the regulations governing the implementation of Section 75 of the Act, passed after heated debate in both houses of parliament in the spring of 2013, just before the Act took effect. As a result CCGs have to put any services due for contractual renewal out to formal tender in the market place, unless the CCG can prove there is only one provider capable of delivering the service. Since it is virtually impossible to prove this to everyone's satisfaction, most CCGs believe that almost all services now have to go through the lengthy, tedious, expensive and bureaucratic formal NHS tender process.

What's more, CCGs are fearful of challenges from the private sector if contracts are not put out to tender, challenges which could involve considerable legal costs which CCGs can scarcely afford. An example of such a challenge to the NHS by a private company came in Blackpool in 2013. The local private hospital is owned by Spire,* who accused the local CCG of 'anti-competitive' behaviour when it failed to offer patients the choice of Spire's private hospital as well as the local foundation trust. Spire was aggrieved that a 'block contract' seemed to direct patients towards the NHS hospital.

It took Monitor a full year to investigate the accusation (though surprisingly they never spoke to any patients, GPs or practice managers in that time).[23] The lengthy and costly investigation eventually found that the CCG had not acted in contravention of the section 75 rules but insisted that in future the CCG should 'promote choice' more openly when patients were offered their first outpatient appointment.[24] Time, energy and public funds had been wasted to satisfy the demands of the English healthcare market. If Spire had not been allowed to make the accusation, more NHS resources could have been spent on patient care rather than seeking to increase Spire's £100m annual income.

* A company formed in 2007 when BUPA sold their hospitals to Cinven, a private equity firm. Spire's net income in 2013 was £99.7m.

Up to now the only CCG to have tested out Lansley's promise that they would not have to open up a tender for services has been the country's largest: North, East and West Devon. Its decisions have not been without controversy (primarily because of their award of part of a contract to a social enterprise) but there has been no wasteful and costly tendering process.[25] With some CCGs already admitting their reluctance to act against failing contractors for fear of legal action,[26] it remains to be seen if any others will have the courage to stand up in defence of services rather than cower before the calls for competition and the threat of legal challenges from the private sector.

Riding roughshod over local decisions

Lansley promised that GPs would make decisions about local services, along with local people, but the example of Lewisham – discussed in Chapter 6 – proved him to be a liar yet again. Local GPs and the CCG completely opposed the proposed downgrading of the hospital, but despite all Lansley's fine words of reassurance, professional views were ignored (along with the views of tens of thousands of locals who took to the streets in protest). Lansley's successor, Jeremy Hunt, attempted to force the changes through, and only High Court legal action stopped the proposed closures and downgrade going ahead. The whole episode showed how little real influence CCGs have when their decisions are unwelcome to the government, and exposed the myth that GPs would be in control as a result of the HSC Act.

Having lost the battle in the High Court Jeremy Hunt then pushed through a law that would prevent future 'Lewisham defeats'. This was to be done by inserting a new Clause 118 (since renumbered 119) into the otherwise unrelated Care

Bill. This is now better known as the 'hospital closure' clause. It gave a Trust Special Administrator powers to impose arbitrary closures anywhere in the general vicinity of what was branded a 'failing' hospital trust. It meant no area of the country could feel safe from the threat of a possible closure of local services.[27]

As the journalist Benedict Cooper wrote in the *New Statesman*, Hunt 'presses ahead Thatcher-like, wilfully ignorant, skipping around every tiresome obstacle, using new tools like Clause 118 to take more power and control away from the people who have paid for the NHS and who need it the most'.[28] Hunt's new piece of legislation means that GPs (and CCGs) are most certainly not in control when it comes to imposing controversial closures; all power would be in the hands of a Special Administrator, appointed by the Secretary of State.

The clause was a spiteful act which demonstrated a profound contempt for previous promises about giving power to patients and doctors. Local GPs' views were ignored by the TSA in Lewisham – while hospital consultants are effectively excluded from almost all aspects of decision-making by the new system.

It's worth noting that passage of this legislation again relied on the Liberal Democrats, who once more trotted obediently through the government lobby to vote with the Tories. Indeed Lib Dem MP Paul Burstow put the final nail in the coffin at the last minute by withdrawing his amendment, which would have allowed local commissioners to have the final say.[29] Voters must not be allowed to forget how the Liberal Democrats repeatedly betrayed the NHS between 2010 and 2015.

A force to be reckoned with?

One of the new organisations that purports to represent CCGs is NHS Clinical Commissioners (NHSCC).[30] It claims that over 85 per cent of CCGs are members and boasts that it meets regularly with NHS England, the Secretary of State for Health, DoH, Monitor, CQC, TDA, NICE and others to raise the issues that might be holding commissioners back and help to find solutions and shape national policy.

Function of NHS Clinical Commissioners[31]

The NHS Commissioning Assembly and NHS Clinical Commissioners work in partnership in supporting the development of the commissioning system. As the community of all commissioning leaders, the NHS Commissioning Assembly acts as the key vehicle to enable NHS England and CCGs to work together on national issues. It works on the premise that as commissioners, NHS England and CCGs, will achieve more together than apart and that collectively we should develop, share and implement solutions focused on the biggest issues where commissioners together have most impact. As the independent voice of CCGs at a national level, NHS Clinical Commissioners influences policy development and implementation and acts as a critical friend to all relevant national bodies (including NHS England and other Arms Lengths Bodies, like Monitor and NTDA [National Trust Development Authority], patient and professional representative groups and government) on CCG issues and on the environment.

By working together, the NHS Commissioning Assembly and NHS Clinical Commissioners have an opportunity to coproduce solutions which help us all work more effectively in the interests of patients.

The membership of the NHSCC Board gives a clue as to the background and agenda of the organisation. Some names crop up that have been around for a while[32] and include

- Dr Shane Gordon – famous for championing the HSC Bill before Parliament's Public Accounts Committee in 2011 and lead author of a letter in support of the Bill when it was running into trouble. His 'leadership' was gratefully acknowledged by Andrew Lansley in Parliament. Dr Gordon is now leading a major initiative to outsource commissioning work in his local North East Essex CCG with a single 'lead provider' charged with commissioning and coordinating 'care closer to home'.[33]
- Dr Michael Dixon – chair of a government friendly organisation, NHS Alliance. Former advisor to Lord Darzi.
- Dr Charles Alessi – chair of another government friendly organisation, National Association of Primary Care.*
- Dr Jonny Marshall – has trodden the corridors of power for many years and helped to found NHSCC. He was rewarded for his loyalty by being made an advisor to the NHS Commissioning Board Executive Team in 2012 'supporting their work on the future design of the NHS'. He was also appointed as policy director for the NHS Confederation – an organisation that receives large sums of money from the Department of Health while its democratic processes remain clouded in secrecy.

With these government friendly GPs on board the NHSCC punches above its weight with plenty of press coverage and an ability to open doors in Whitehall for conversations over NHS policy. The BMA General Practitioners Committee

* Both Dixon and Alessi were cheerleaders for Lansley's Bill.

should be negotiating on behalf of GPs but see that much of their representative and negotiating powers are seeping away to the NHSCC.

Health and Wellbeing Boards, and Co-commissioning

In other unsettling news Labour's shadow health secretary Andy Burnham has proposed that if they win power in 2015 he will give control of commissioning to Health and Wellbeing Boards that are run by London boroughs, county and unitary councils.[34] This has been met with widespread concern given the continual reduction in councils' budgets and contribution to social care, and the failure of Health and Wellbeing Boards to establish any significant profile or independence. GPs in particular have for over 100 years been suspicious of and resisted any control over them by local councils: they are unlikely to respond any more favourably to such proposals from a Labour government.

The latest idea from the coalition government is called 'co-commissioning'.[35] NHS England is devolving more work down to already hard pressed CCGs as they realise that Local Area Teams are too short staffed to undertake their work effectively. It is proposed that CCGs will take on the day-to-day management of GP contracts and performance manage the payments to practices and the services they offer. GPs will have even less influence and control with co-commissioning because those who sit on a CCG would have to remove themselves from the room when any discussions take place on GP contracts and payments control. There is also a serious risk that any GPs on CCGs who performance manage their colleagues will be seen as part of the NHS system 'doing bad things' to general practice. This could rapidly eroded what little trust there is between GP CCG leaders and grass-roots GPs.

The failure of the BMA

How did GPs in particular and medical professionals in general end up as the victims of legislation that promised so much and delivered so little? One of the most powerful and prominent organisations which Lansley managed to neutralise was the British Medical Association (BMA). The BMA is the main medical trades union, representing 147,000 of the UK's 250,000 registered doctors, and thus had an influential role in advising doctors whether to support or oppose government 'reforms'. Within the BMA the General Practitioners Committee (GPC) represents the UK's 40,000 GPs.

The BMA leaders failed to recognise the dangers inherent in the Lansley Bill and wasted months when they should have been campaigning against it pursuing a policy of 'critical engagement'. This achieved nothing apart from allowing Lansley to claim that doctors backed the reforms, a claim he repeated unchallenged up to and including the day the legislation passed.

The BMA and the HSC Bill

Despite the fact that the HSC Bill contained sweeping changes, neither the British Medical Association (BMA), the main trade union representing doctors, nor its General Practitioners Committee were willing to consult English doctors about their views on the proposed changes.

Their paternalistic attitude was summed up by the then GP leader, Dr Laurence Buckman: 'we know what they think, we don't need to survey them'. As a result many doctors felt let down by the BMA, which failed to voice their hostility to the HSC Bill. However, surveys of GP opinion by *Pulse* magazine and by the professional body, the Royal College of General Practitioners, showed time and again that a majority of GPs were against the Bill. Had their opposition been given public expression in a refusal to engage with the process, it would have made it extremely difficult for Lansley and Cameron to push the Bill through.

This lack of professional leadership from the BMA was compounded by the fact that much of the media, in particular the BBC, obediently regurgitated the coalition line that the legislation was about 'giving more power to GPs and to patients'. This played into the government's hands and allowed them to bulldoze through one of the most undemocratic Acts of recent parliamentary history with little public awareness of what the implications would be.[36]

There were serious concerns over the professional implications of rationing care and some GPs were anxious that the General Medical Council (GMC) might take a dim view if they refused to refer patients on to hospitals.* West Sussex GP Jerry Luke received huge support at an annual BMA conference for his resolution calling on the General Medical Council to 'reaffirm that commissioning GPs' primary responsibility is to their patients, not to financial balance'. At the conference, Luke warned:

* Ironically at the same time that GPs were being asked to restrict hospital referrals by their CCGs they were being blamed by politicians and the national press for failing to diagnose cancer at an early stage – which almost always requires hospital investigations – and encouraged by NICE to increase their referral rates. http://www.bbc.com/news/health-30119230; http://www.mirror.co.uk/news/uk-news/gps-failing-thousands-cancer-patients-2899973.

> I fear that without the GMC telling us our patients have to come first – before the money – we are going to be led by some of our colleagues who are quite happy to cut and slash just like the Department of Health wants. I personally am not prepared to carry on like this. I've been up close and personal to the decisions CCGs have to make. They have only one real duty, and that is to end the year in budget. Everything else is secondary to that. You'll hear from the advocates of clinical commissioning that it is outcome focused and clinically appropriate. Do not be seduced by snake oil salesmen. CCGs can run out of services, but they must not run out of money.[37]

The BMA's failures – either to consult their members or to understand the Bill – allowed Lansley to get away with his legislation. Why didn't the BMA leaders – in particular Dr Hamish Meldrum and Dr Laurence Buckman, both GPs themselves – heed repeated calls to survey their members? Perhaps they were frightened of the answer, afraid that doctors might oppose the Bill and thus drag the BMA out of the corridors of power and make it fight for its members. Whatever the reason it was a critical mistake by the BMA and the consequences will be felt for years.

Professor Clare Gerada (then chair of the Royal College of General Practitioners – RCGP) was an exception amongst GP leaders. She was not afraid to oppose the coalition health reforms, although she later admitted that her ardent campaigning had made her ill.[38] In her final keynote speech to her College she said 'in ten years' time, I predict, the NHS Act will be viewed as one of the historic misjudgements of all time'.[39]

In 2014 the RCGP launched a clever and high profile campaigning strategy 'Put Patients First – back general practice'.[40] It focused on the recruitment and retention crisis in general practice and successfully highlighted the reduction in funding for primary care. Many commentators took notice and the campaign attracted much media coverage. Campaigning is territory that BMA used to effectively own but in recent years their GP committee seems to prefer contemplating its own navel rather than send out the message that general practice was on the verge of destruction.*

Morale and recruitment

The 2010 coalition government has overseen an unprecedented collapse in morale in general practice. Dr Maureen Baker, the new leader of the Royal College of General Practitioners, warned in 2014 that general practice is on the 'brink of extinction'.[41] There have been year on year cuts in the share of NHS spending for general practice, and the RCGP estimates real terms budgets will have fallen by 17 per cent by 2017.[42] Meanwhile the government, pointing to the £2.5bn a year increases to the NHS to keep pace with price inflation, claims that they have increased the NHS budget.[43] In five years of flatline real terms funding, primary care, together with mental health, has suffered actual cuts.

The increasing financial pressures and unmanageable workload are causing GPs to run for the hills and retire early.[44] In one 2014 survey, a shocking six out of ten GPs

---

* Perhaps the fact that the average age of GPC committee membership was over fifty, with retirement and a good pension pot beckoning, meant they preferred not rock the boat. Younger members of the profession must have wondered why there was such a deafening silence from GPC HQ.

were considering retiring early due to the pressures and to constant denigration of the profession.[45] Norfolk based GP Dr John Harris-Hall said of his decision to retire early:

The increasing demand and workload pressure are leading to low morale and stress, causing many GPs like myself to leave the profession. I am sad to retire early but I feel there is no other choice. Enough is enough.[46]

Not surprisingly young doctors considering their future careers are not attracted by general practice. Consequently there is a looming recruitment crisis, and in 2014 – for the first time ever – NHS leaders were scrabbling around trying to find more doctors willing to train to become GPs. Dr Krishna Kasaraneni, former chair of the BMA's trainee GP subcommittee, said it was unlikely that an attempt to find further recruits would dramatically improve uptake or cover the shortfall of new trainees.[47] The lack of new recruits to general practice combined with the early retirement of thousands of GPs has the makings of a perfect storm in primary care, with far fewer GPs than are needed to see the patients in our communities.

In October 2014 alarm bells even began to ring for ministers and Jeremy Hunt hastily announced an independent review to establish how many GPs would be needed in the future.[48] Handily for Mr Hunt the review would not report until after the 2015 general election, leading many to accuse him of kicking the issue into the long grass in order to avoid difficult questions in the run-up to polling day. The BMA welcomed the review[49] but many felt it was too little too late as the profession was already on its knees.

Despite the belated review, battles over plans that would

severely cut or eliminate the special funding for some GP practices in deprived areas have again pointed up the inequality of access to GP services, which could be made worse if some of the affected practices are closed. In November 2014 *Pulse* magazine published a survey suggesting that as a result of this threat one in twenty GPs were thinking of closing their practice in 2015.[50] And this is happening at a time when the political pressure is to push care out into 'the community', resulting in more work for already beleaguered GPs. One could be forgiven for thinking that the politicians are setting primary care up to fail.

The future for general practice

English general practice is in crisis, its workforce demoralised by political changes and cuts to funding, increased responsibilities, increased pressure and an ever-lengthening working day. The massive top down reorganisation forced on the profession in England (which does not apply to Wales, Scotland or Northern Ireland) has left GPs in the devolved nations standing by in horrified amazement, hoping that such policies are never introduced in their part of the UK.

GPs need strong leaders to represent them and stand up to the politicians and those parts of the media which day in day out seem to be trying to diminish their profession, rundown the NHS, and demoralise them even further.

General practice has been called the 'jewel in the crown' of the NHS. Our system of primary care, acting as the gate keeper to expensive specialist care, is in large part responsible for the efficiency and cost-effectiveness of the service. It would be an act of the utmost folly to undermine it: yet this coalition has done its best to do so. In a few short years the government and Lansley's legislation have combined to destroy GP morale, impose draconian cuts, slash recruitment and push experienced GPs to either resign from the NHS or retire earlier than planned. It's not a record to be proud of – and certainly not what Lansley and Cameron promised GPs and their patients.

5

Myth: Our NHS reforms will reduce bureaucracy and save money.

We are abolishing needless bureaucracy, and our plans will save one third of all administration costs during this Parliament.

Department of Health, 6 September 2011[1]

A Department of Health spokesperson said: 'Our bureaucracy-busting reforms put power in the hands of local doctors and nurses and are saving the NHS over £1bn a year. There are now nearly 7,000 fewer managers and over 16,450 more clinicians than in 2010.'

The Guardian, 26 July 2014[2]

Andrew Lansley promised that his reforms would reduce the NHS bureaucracy that was holding back good patient care. In fact the layers of bureaucracy have increased as a result of the Health and Social Care Act. 150 Primary Care Trusts have become 211 Clinical Commissioning Groups, much of whose onerous work has to be done by Commissioning Support Units, themselves due to be outsourced in 2016. Many other new bodies have been created including NHS England (employing 4,000 people and which in turn has 27 Local Area Teams), Clinical Senates, and others too numerous to mention. As a result lines of accountability have become so complex that the RCGP described them as looking like 'spaghetti junction'.

Lansley also promised that his reforms would save money but this is manifestly untrue. Implementing the reforms is estimated to have cost at least £3bn even before account is taken of their effects. The proportion of the NHS budget spent on administration has risen inexorably as the NHS is marketised, increasing from about 6 per cent before the introduction of Thatcher's internal market to an estimated 15 per cent now. As well as the direct costs of running a market there are the opportunity costs in terms of both money and clinical time which would be better spent on direct patient care rather than on dealing with the demands of a competitive NHS. Despite promises to the contrary the Treasury has clawed back about £5bn from the NHS budget at a time when care is being rationed and waiting lists are growing.

The Health and Social Care Act has increased bureaucracy and complicated lines of accountability. It has wasted money on an unnecessary set of reforms and on establishing and encouraging an NHS market at a time when financial constraints mean that it is imperative not to squander the NHS budget.

* * *

One of the reasons given for the massive reorganisation introduced by Lansley's 'reforms' was to reduce NHS bureaucracy and NHS costs. Lansley claimed that bureaucratic red tape was stopping clinical staff from delivering high quality care and that the Health and Social Care Act would mean fewer layers of management. This 'delayering' would in turn result in savings for the NHS allowing more money for frontline care. In 2009, while still shadow secretary for health, he told a conference in Manchester that a third could be shaved off the annual £4.5bn cost of quangos and NHS management in England.[3] In 2010 he pledged to cut £1bn a year from 'central bureaucracy' and promised that the savings, equivalent to the salaries of more than 30,000 nurses, would be reinvested* in frontline services.[4]

But Professor John Appleby, chief economist at the King's Fund predicted that 'the sheer number of changes being made to the health system as a result of the government's reforms risk creating additional bureaucracy'.[5] The King's Fund thought that the legislation would result in a picture of 'considerable complexity' which would be challenging for health professionals working within it and for patients trying to navigate it,** in other words, a far cry from the simplified system Lansley was promising. Their comment is worth quoting in full:

---

* Another broken promise. It is estimated that the Treasury has clawed back over £5bn from the NHS under the coalition. The NHS has currently 6,000 fewer nurses than when the coalition came to power.
** It is well worth watching their short animation (http://vimeo.com/69224754) on the Byzantine structure of Lansley's new 'streamlined' NHS, illustrating as it does the very 'alphabeti spaghetti' that Cameron promised he would get rid of in a pre-election speech to the RCN (See https://www.youtube.com/watch?v=nH2EmVGowCk.).

The NHS system has grown exponentially, with complex structures developing to underpin it. While there was once a simple accountability hierarchy from front-line services to the Secretary of State, there is now a complex system of public and private providers, with a plethora of regulators who impact on what managers need to do. The advent of the internal market in particular, together with a growing recognition of national and international competition law, means the task is one of complex system management rather than simple administration.[6]

While Strategic Health Authorities and Primary Care Trusts were indeed replaced by a single layer of about 200 Clinical Commissioning Groups (CCGs), these CCGs were faced with the immense task of purchasing services for their patients in an aggressively competitive NHS where the government's new legislation appeared to require compulsory tendering. Most GPs and their colleagues on CCGs had little or no experience in this new role and needed help. Technical advice was to be provided via Commissioning Support Units and help with specialist commissioning would come from Clinical Senates, two entirely new structures.

NHS England (NHSE), the NHS central command and control and yet another new structure, was initially predicted to be 'small and lithe' but already its responsibilities run to many pages. It employs 4,000 people, (until recently 5,500) and has four regional offices as well as 27 local area teams (LATS). Other bodies have sprung up like mushrooms and the Royal College of General Practitioners estimated that the number of NHS statutory bodies was set to climb from 163 to 521 with the lines of accountability looking like 'spaghetti junction'.[7]

Sacked and rehired

Lansley had promised to get rid of NHS managers but he had perhaps overlooked the fact that managers would be needed to help with the complex new structure of the NHS. (The alternative would be to take clinical staff away from frontline care, which of course has happened anyway as CCGs and competitive tendering eat up clinical time). The result was that experienced NHS managers were sacked and then had to be rehired as the government woke up to the fact that good managers were needed to support clinical staff during the introduction of the new legislation.

This failure to anticipate the need for experienced managers was very costly. In July 2014 the *Observer* reported[8] Department of Health figures showing that the cost of redundancy payments for NHS managers had reached almost £1.6bn as a result of the new legislation. The total included compensation paid to some 4,000 'revolving door' managers, who left after May 2010 with large pay-outs and then returned either on full-time or part-time contracts.* Cutting managers is also proving to be a false economy.

Cutting costs – quite the contrary

Along with his claims about cutting layers of management Lansley also said that his HSC Act would result in savings, another promise which fails to stand up to scrutiny. The cost of the reorganisation alone was predicted to be between £1bn and £3bn but as we have seen at least £1.6bn has already

---

* The figures showed that in 2013-14 a total of 6,330 'exit packages' were agreed for NHS staff, at a cost of £197m. This took the total since 2010-11, when the government launched its reform plans, to 38,419 packages totalling £1.588bn. In 2013, 237 managers received payoffs of between £100,000 and £150,000, 83 of between £150,000 and £200,000, and 40 of over £200,000.

been spent on redundancies, and many of these staff have had to be re-employed at further expense. This is only a small part of the costs incurred by the Act.

Reinforcing the NHS market through policies such as competitive tendering brings its own significant costs, including the costs of the tenders themselves, plus all the paraphernalia of the market including management consultants, lawyers and accountants, not to mention the very real cost of the time spent by clinical staff away from their patients.

Governments have always been shy about the cost of the NHS market in England, (discussed at greater length in Chapter 2) and have profited from useful confusions between the cost of administering the NHS and the cost of managing it.[9] (It is these semantic muddles that allow MPs to stand up in the House of Commons and make contrary claims about the NHS while quite convinced that each is correct). It has been estimated that the NHS market has taken administration costs from approximately 6 per cent of the English NHS budget to somewhere in the region of 15 per cent, meaning that at the most conservative estimate it costs an additional £5-10bn a year to run the English NHS as a competitive market.[10] Since Lansley's reforms ramped up the market through competitive tendering and full on competition, overseen by Monitor, it is inevitable that the costs have gone up. The government is not of course telling us anything, but there have been noticeably few claims for cost savings after Lansley's original promise.

The minimum estimate of £5bn currently wasted on pointless market activities would fund both the £4bn annual increase in NHS spending (needed to keep pace with pressures on the service) with some left over to contribute to free critical social care for everyone who needs it, which the King's Fund's Barker Commission recently said would cost 'substantially less' than £3bn a year. But the whole subject of the cost, purpose and value of a market in health care is an evidence free zone in which politicians make unsubstantiated claims that – if they were doctors – would have had them struck off or welcomed as snake oil salesmen years ago. Almost all so-called think tanks have also avoided the subject like the plague, perhaps concerned that government funding (for example over £500,000 since 2010 for the King's Fund)[11] might dry up if they pointed out the obvious fact that the savings from abandoning an unwanted market would go a long way to filling funding gaps.

True to form the coalition government simply turned a blind eye to the additional costs of their expanding market or lied about them. For example the impact assessment for the contentious section 75 regulations (which introduced competitive tendering and were signed off by the ever reassuring Earl Howe) even went so far as to claim that with competitive tendering 'there are negligible direct costs to patients, commissioners or providers'.[12] David Lock QC wrote in an angry blog:

> That statement would be laughable if this were not so serious. Another part of government, the Cabinet Office, has recognised the huge costs of procurement exercises and is complaining that too much cost is imposed by these exercises. This appears to be another case of a total absence of joined up government.

He added:

Procurement processes are hugely expensive and they delay contracts for extended periods. Conservative MPs ought to have learned that from the West Coast Rail tendering debacle which left the Department of Transport with a bill of £50m when just one tender exercise went wrong. These Regulations will impose countless procurement competitions on the NHS, and cause vast resources to move from patient care into administration.[13]

While we have heard very little about savings arising from the HSC Act, some alarming facts have come to light about the costs of the NHS market. The expense involved in the tendering process – a scandalous waste of public money according to one senior NHS manager[14] – are discussed in Chapter 10. Suffice it to say here that a recent tendering process in Cambridgeshire (eventually awarded to a local NHS consortium) cost £1m, money which a cash strapped NHS can hardly afford to waste on bidding for its own services.

In 2013 a FoI request to CCGs revealed that they had spent over £5m on competition lawyers in the six months following the introduction of competitive tendering. This figure did not include similar expenses for NHS hospitals and NHS providers forced to tender for their own services. Labour, who had discovered the figure, estimated that this was equivalent to the cost of over 5,670 cataract operations, 873 knee operations or 841 hip replacements at a time when these treatments were being rationed.[15]

At the same time Labour reported a survey showing that nine out of ten hospital leaders wanted the incoming NHS chief executive to make removal of competition regulations his top priority.[16] Not surprising, as it has been hard to find supporters of the NHS market anywhere beyond the major political parties and those health professionals and NHS watchers who see their star rising as they promote what the government wants to hear.

Management consultants or medical consultants?

Another area where costs have risen despite reassurances to the contrary from Andrew Lansley is the money lavished on management consultants. After the election Lansley claimed to be 'staggered by the scale of the expenditure on management consultants', which stood at £313m in 2010, and promised to slash it. But after four years of coalition government the costs had doubled to £640m a year, almost £1.8m per day and enough to hire an extra 20,000 nurses or run three medium sized hospitals.[17] David Oliver, formerly of the DoH, blamed the health reforms for this explosion, pointing out that racketeers profit in times of chaos. Rumours circulated that senior management consultants were being paid £4,000 per day and that Monitor (largely staffed by ex-employees of management consultants) was spending an eye watering £32m on management consultancy firms (Oliver noted that only seven of Monitor's 337 employees had any frontline clinical experience). The *BMJ* article is worth reading as an example of profligate spending by people who claim that we can't afford the NHS.[18] One thing is sure – the public would rather see their taxes spent on medical not management consultants. Once again they aren't being given the choice.

Conclusion

The concern of the NHS Confederation that the HSC Act would lead to a 'tsunami of bureaucracy' proved well founded.[19] The Act has resulted in a worse bureaucratic tangle, with more layers of management resulting in increased spending on administration. In 2013 Jeremy Hunt called on the NHS Confederation to review the problem of bureaucracy, thus tacitly admitting that the HSC Act had not delivered on its promise. Their review found that 40 per cent of clinicians and NHS managers spent between one and three hours a day collecting and recording information, with 75 per cent feeling that certain information they were asked to provide was irrelevant. It reported that the average doctor and nurse spent ten hours a week on bureaucracy, more than a quarter of their working week and a truly shocking statistic when there is a chronic shortage of frontline staff to care for patients. And tellingly the review suggested that the blame lay at least in part with Lansley's reorganisation of the NHS, with 'a lack of clarity of roles and responsibilities resulting in duplicated requests' for information and data.[20]

At the same time a survey by the RCN found that nurses were 'drowning in paperwork' including filing, photocopying and ordering supplies.[21] It is difficult to avoid the conclusion that if Lansley had paid more attention to helping clinical staff do the work they were trained to do rather than requiring them to write bids for their own services and fill in forms then the NHS and its patients would be in much better shape today.

Lansley's 'reforms' have incurred further costs associated with an expanding commercial market for the English NHS. Lansley's promises about reduced bureaucracy and lower costs have proved as empty as the NHS coffers under the coalition government.

6

Myth: Our NHS reforms will give more power and voice to local people.

There will be no decision about you without you.[1]

One of the things we are intending to do is create much greater opportunities for patients' voices to be heard.[2]

Andrew Lansley

Andrew Lansley and David Cameron repeatedly promised that the Health and Social Care Act would give greater powers to patients and a louder voice to local communities when it came to health matters. The reality is that the patient voice is fainter than ever as the organisations representing patients become weaker, 'consultations' become more of a sham and NHS bodies become more secretive.

The patient voice was strongest when represented by Community Health Councils (CHCs). CHCs could and did visit and report on local NHS services, organise local campaigns and hold NHS bureaucrats to account. They were abolished by Alan Milburn in 2003, and replaced by a succession of weak bodies culminating in Healthwatch, established by the HSC Act.

Real patient voice has become politically inconvenient as more NHS 'reforms' have been pushed through against the wishes of the public. 'Consultations' are held at short notice or not at all, and any findings are likely to be misrepresented or shelved if unhelpful. The public and the press have more difficulty finding out what is being done in their name as new NHS bodies hold meetings out of the public eye and are not obliged to publish minutes. The private sector is able to hide its profits and outcomes behind commercial confidentiality.

The more political rhetoric there has been about patient voice the less genuine engagement there has been with the public. The proliferation of local NHS campaigns and action groups is an indication of the fact that many people feel that legitimate avenues of enquiry and complaint have been closed to them, leaving little option but to take to the streets in order to be heard.

* * *

In the run-up to the 2010 general election, David Cameron and his shadow health secretary Andrew Lansley repeatedly promised to protect the NHS from local cutbacks and reconfiguration, but also to give increased public voice and control over local services.[3]

As soon as he had taken office, Lansley repeated similar pledges. At the 2010 conference of the NHS employers' body the NHS Confederation Lansley insisted:

> As we set out in the coalition agreement, for the first time the voice of the public will be heard across commissioning, the public health service and social care. In these straitened financial times this accountability for how we use taxpayers' money is even more important.[4]

However, this commitment, like the promise to halt closures of A&E and maternity units and deliver a real terms increase in NHS spending each year, proved to be worthless.

The Tories' overriding commitment to 'austerity' policies* to address the immense hole in government finances created by the multi-billion bail-out of the banks. This meant that local policies have, since 2010, had to be shaped not around the 'voice of the public' but around the drive for cost-cutting 'reconfiguration' of hospital and other services – driving through unpopular cuts regardless of local opinion.

As a result even the limited avenues for local communities to register their concerns on local schemes and plans have

---

* A policy which the IMF has now decided was a big mistake – see Mayeda, A. 2014. 'IMF's Post-Crisis Austerity Call Mistaken, Watchdog Says', Bloomberg, 4 November 2014: http://www.bloomberg.com/news/2014-11-04/imf-s-post-crisis-austerity-call-mistaken-watchdog-says.html?hootPostID=913aee1114adb25290ac384f63ae0f80.

been further restricted or closed off. New, even less forceful and representative local bodies have been set up by Lansley's Health and Social Care Act – bodies that have played little or no role in defending any of the threatened hospitals and services, and which few people even know exist.

The result has been a serious and growing problem in which not only the public's views but also their legitimate concerns over the viability of proposals and the knock-on impact they are likely to have on other services are effectively excluded from final decision-making and from any later review of decisions that have been made. Campaigners – lacking any regular democratic access to express their views – are obliged to resort to street protests and petitions, or to judicial review in which only the legal process itself is ever scrutinised, not the merits of the proposals that have been put forward.

The report of the People's Inquiry into London's NHS also sums up the situation in many other parts of the country, when it points out:

> In every part of London we have heard an overwhelming sense of frustration at the lack, or inadequacy, of channels for public engagement with many commissioners and provider trusts. We have seen little evidence of public or professional confidence in the official box-ticking consultation processes. There is equally little evidence that commissioners or providers give serious consideration or in some cases respond at all to issues and doubts raised during consultation exercises.[5]

The gagging of the public voice

The problem is worse than ever, but not new. For the past thirty years or more NHS 'consultations' have often been seen as little more than a pointless ritual, designed to blow off steam while eventually allowing unelected NHS managers to force through most of the changes they want regardless of local community views and wishes. Any real power was not in the consultation process itself, but in the various mechanisms through which the public could get information on what was being proposed, and organisations representing the public could intervene to delay or even stop some of the most controversial changes.

But more recently even these standby mechanisms have been undermined – while governments, health bosses and civil servants give empty promises to enhance the voice of local people. The last fifteen years have seen the abolition of the statutory bodies which once gave local people much more influence – and the ability to halt controversial changes pending a ministerial decision. Since 2000 the proliferation of private and confidential contracts and tendering processes has led to increased secrecy due to 'commercial confidentiality'. This has reduced the public's right even to know what is being proposed by local health commissioners – and to develop a coherent critique and response to plans which many would oppose if they knew of them.

Some of the most contested policies arising from Labour's 2000 NHS Plan were negotiated by Department of Health officials at national level, and then imposed on local commissioners whether they liked it or not – most notably the early contracts for Independent Sector Treatment Centres and diagnostic services.[6] Other plans were hatched up in the early 2000s by the newly-created Commercial Directorate, charged with creating a new competitive market in elective care behind the closed doors of Whitehall and away from any public scrutiny.[7]

An even more authoritarian approach has developed recently taking advantage of the Unsustainable Provider Regime established by New Labour. This sets out the precise and rigid timetable for the intervention of a government-appointed Trust Special Administrator with draconian powers to intervene where a trust or foundation trust is seen as 'failing'.[8] This has been followed in the last two years by the Tory-led coalition taking extraordinary steps to add a new Clause 119 to the HSC Act that gives even more sweeping powers to close hospitals, where necessary against the wishes of local people, even when the hospitals under the axe are not the ones in financial difficulties.[9]

There has seldom been more official rhetoric about 'engagement' with patients and the local public and less actual engagement with anything other than supportive views. This rhetoric stands in stark contrast to those Clinical Commissioning Groups (CCGs) – such as Bedfordshire, Cambridgeshire and several in Staffordshire – who have been taking legal advice on how best to phrase their refusal to consult local people on controversial changes, or publish even basic documents and general information on what they are doing or the contracts they are asking NHS and private sector providers to bid for.

How it was: the heyday of the Community Health Councils

The biggest blow against any public voice on major change in the NHS was the abolition of Community Health Councils (CHCs). Up until then, especially in the final few years of John Major's government and the first few years of Tony Blair's

New Labour, some of the best and most proactive Community Health Councils had been at the peak of their effectiveness.

CHCs had been set up in 1974 as statutory bodies, independently funded through regional health authorities, with a brief to represent patients and the local public. Most CHCs included an elected component representing local communities, charities and other organisations. With full time staff, the best CHCs developed a body of expertise, and a group of local activists and experts who knew the structure and working of local services, could champion patient complaints and give voice to their concerns, and were empowered to visit hospital wards and clinics.[10] They were able to report and register their views through representation on the boards of health authorities. A strong CHC could strike fear into the hearts of many NHS bureaucrats and senior staff – and could also rally local public support when a more substantial issue arose.

Beginning from an initiative in Southwark monitoring the A&E at King's College Hospital, a network of over 150 CHCs in England (and Wales prior to devolution in 1999) developed, and conducted regular coordinated monitoring of delays and issues in A&E departments, publishing devastating reports which grabbed press headlines.[11]

Some local campaigns were very powerful. In North London, Barnet CHC was a was willing throughout to support one of the most massive and wide-reaching campaigns, which from 1995 fought to stop the closure of Edgware Hospital, whose catchment straddled three boroughs, Barnet, Brent and Harrow – and included a number of marginal constituencies. The Edgware Hospital campaign held huge meetings, lobbies, demonstrations – and won support from almost every organisation in the area, from the Brent Cross traders and local businesses through every religious and ethnic community.

The campaign successfully pressurised one local Tory, Sir John Gorst, to break the whip of the struggling Major government, in order to press the campaign to keep the hospital open. He and a number of other Tory MPs subsequently lost their seats in 1997, while New Labour, having gained politically from the campaign, proceeded rapidly and shamelessly to close down the remaining services at Edgware that people had fought so hard to keep.

Soon after the 1997 election another local CHC was also right at the centre of a huge campaign, this time to defend Kidderminster Hospital, a fight which eventually cost the sitting Labour MP David Lock his seat after he backed its closure. Over 50,000 people marched through the small town of Kidderminster, and large numbers packed consultation meetings. The local Wyre Forest council joined with the CHC to challenge plans for the closure of 200 beds, A&E and most acute services at what had been a top performing hospital, and councillors from all parties voted unanimously to back a detailed document arguing the case against the closure.[12]

However all of this was simply ignored by the District Health Authority. They even confronted a judicial review, and went shamelessly into court where they found a judge who would uphold their right not to answer any of the vital questions raised by local elected bodies about the viability of services and finances if the closure went ahead. The DHA pressed ahead with their flawed plan for a new PFI Hospital in Worcester which, as campaigners had predicted, went badly wrong, with beds in seriously short supply, the promised efficiencies and shorter lengths of stay failing to materialise, and the extra costs of PFI pushing the trust into long-running financial problems.

These were just a couple of the many fiercely independent CHCs which spoke up for local communities and patients up and down the country. It was these campaigners who incurred the wrath of ministers rather than the handful of deadbeat CHCs which allowed local NHS managers to call the shots.

Foundations erode democracy

The onslaught on the public voice has escalated in parallel with the creation of a competitive market in health care from 2001 onwards. Then, with the Labour Party still smarting from the recent loss of a sitting MP in Kidderminster in the 2001 election, Health Secretary Alan Milburn brought in proposals to scrap CHCs in England in the same legislation that established foundation trusts (in 2003) as part of the 2000 NHS Plan. Market style healthcare systems and reforms appear to be incompatible with even the relative modicum of local accountability and voice that prevailed at the time of the Kidderminster hospital campaign.

So CHCs were to be silenced, and replaced with the first of a confusing succession of toothless and largely neglected new bodies which few people ever heard of or understood (the most recent version of which is Healthwatch, established by the Health and Social Care Act).

It is no coincidence that the suppression of the public's voice through CHCs came alongside the establishment of foundation trusts: one of their more frequently exercised 'freedoms' was that they were no longer required to meet in public or publish their board papers – or significant information on their performance and finances.[13] Sadly an already tame news media was by then downsizing almost every aspect of local reporting as newsroom staff were cut to boost short-term profits. The media became even more reluctant to carry any detailed coverage of changes taking place in the NHS, and local newspapers and broadcasters raised no complaint at the obstacles that would be erected to prevent journalists obtaining information on the day-to-day business and longer term plans of local trusts.

Transforming community services – into businesses

This erosion of local democracy was followed by the drive from 2005 to 'transform community services', which involved separating them from the Primary Care Trusts which in most cases were delivering these services, while also commissioning hospital and mental health care. Community services were to be separated either into free-standing NHS trusts, or floated off outside the NHS by becoming non-profit 'social enterprises'. Labour went on to establish a 'right to request' in which any group of staff working in community health services could in theory request the opportunity to break away as a 'social enterprise' – although every single incidence of such requests was led not by frontline staff, but by the most senior management.[14]

In those community services that became social enterprises NHS trained staff would find themselves no longer NHS employees or covered by NHS terms and conditions beyond the limited protection of the TUPE regulations for staff transferred. The bodies would be outside the public sector, and run as businesses; the Freedom of Information Act would no longer apply.

Where these changes were implemented, they were carried through with little if any consultation with the local public – and often little or none even with the frontline staff concerned. Among the social enterprises that were set up, some, far from empowering staff, chose instead to derecognise their trade unions. In East of England, a hotbed of privatisation and fragmentation, UNISON noted:

> [S]ix of the 14 PCT provider arms in the six counties and two unitary authorities of Eastern England are seeking to remain within the NHS as Community Foundation Trusts, while the other eight look to wholly or partly non-NHS solutions.[15]

None of them proposed to consult the local public.

The Department of Health set up a whole unit to encourage and advise NHS managers on how to split off their services from the rest of the NHS and its management, and developed a deceptive rhetoric stressing the 'power' that would be given to frontline staff to 'innovate' and improve care for patients.[16]

This of course distracted attention from the fact that these non-profit social enterprises were businesses that would be forced eventually to compete with ruthless for-profit businesses in order to win the contracts they needed to keep them going. It would not be enough for a social enterprise just to break even each year. They had to deliver a surplus to allow any possibility of development: the pressures were hardly different from a private business. Moreover there was little reason why staff, whose views would have been completely ignored in setting up such social enterprises without their agreement, should have any confidence that the same domineering managers would take any note of them once the new business had been set up.

The further step of tendering contracts for various community health services to 'any willing provider' – encouraging the for-profit sector as well as non-profits to slice off the services that seemed most lucrative and risk-free – also began in this same period, again generally with little or no public consultation. This policy was only halted briefly during the tenure of Andy Burnham (Health Secretary from the autumn of 2009 up to the 2010 election), who declared that the NHS should be the 'preferred provider'.[17]

Darzi and consultation

In 2007 NHS London commissioned Lord Darzi's report on health care in the capital, which proposed sweeping changes to the structures of hospitals and primary care services, with the introduction of 'polyclinics' – a policy rejected by the BMA. This was followed by a farcical 'consultation' conducted by NHS London, in which just 3,700 'individuals and organisations' responded (0.07 per cent) from a London electorate of 5.3 million – at a cost of £15m. The average cost per response of over £4,000 would have been enough to fly each respondent to the Bahamas for a focus group.

So the claimed '51 per cent majority' for the Darzi proposals suggests a grand total of less than 1900 Londoners gave any mandate for the plan. (Even this is not clear. The ballot was conducted by Ipsos Mori, the consultants who had previously produced a contorted report on the public's views of the proposed 'Picture of Health' reconfiguration of hospital services in south-east London. This completely sidestepped the evidence of the actual public voice by focusing not on the overwhelming rejection of the key proposals, but instead repeatedly highlighting the 'interesting' views of the tiny minorities that had registered some level of support).[18]

While still a Labour Minister Lord Darzi did however offer an important set of pledges, which if they were ever put into practice would give the public a serious voice and a chance to influence changes. Trying to win back some credibility for the proposals, he offered five promises:

- 'Change will always be to the benefit of patients.'
- 'Change will be clinically driven.'
- 'All change will be locally led.'
- 'You will be involved.'
- 'You will see the difference first. Existing services will not be withdrawn until new and better services are available to patients so they can see the difference.'[19]

The final one is potentially the most far-reaching pledge, since it committed NHS bosses to establishing new and improved services before existing services could be withdrawn and buildings closed. A pledge that no government up to now has been willing to carry out.

New Labour's reorganisation of primary care trusts and strategic health authorities, merging them into larger, less accountable bodies, reduced further the impact of the public voice, but it did at least leave intact a framework of PCTs and SHAs as public bodies meeting in public and publishing the bulk of their board papers.

This was all swept away by the Health and Social Care Act. The CCGs it created are expected to meet in public, but occasionally take decisions behind closed doors. They are expected to publish board papers, but too often resort to claims of 'commercial in confidence' to withhold information on the increasing variety of tendering processes that they have been forced towards by the regulations governing the implementation of section 75 of the Act.

Draconian powers

In 2009 the Unsustainable Provider Regime, giving draconian powers to a Trust Special Administrator (TSA), was introduced by Health Secretary Alan Johnson, and was ready and waiting for the Conservative-led coalition to use when they chose to override local opinion.[20] In the summer of 2013 these powers were invoked for the first time, to address the crisis of the South London Healthcare Trust.[21] The eventual proposals impacted most heavily on Lewisham Hospital. The lion's share of cuts to fund a bail-out of the debt-ridden PFI contracts in South London Healthcare fell on Lewisham, a neighbouring but completely separate trust that was not in deficit or even serving the same catchment.

The hugely restricted 'consultation process' incorporated in the TSA timetable spectacularly failed to take any account of the overwhelming views of the local public, or of health professionals in the hospitals. Lewisham's GPs, who came out clearly against the TSA plan, were also ignored, making a nonsense of claims that GPs were somehow in charge of the newly reorganised NHS.

Guidance for Cynical Commissioning Groups or How to get away with it!

All the guidance you need to turn any popular and successful local general hospital into a clinic – or housing development.

Remember the consultation process is your way of brushing aside popular resistance and informed criticism. So make sure your consultation document is decorated with the full gamut of spurious options and skewed questionnaires giving no chance to say NO to your cuts.

Set up a series of poorly advertised, one-sided meetings for you to rattle on to small audiences at inconvenient times and inaccessible locations. Print inadequate numbers of patchily distributed documents: make sure translations are only of summaries and appear late in the consultation – if at all.

The one thing to remember is never, ever to answer any awkward questions that may be raised or address genuine concerns in your response to the consultation.

That's it! If you follow these simple steps you can gag the opposition and push your plans through. You will be unpopular, of course – but, hey, you will keep your job, even as others lose theirs.

John Lister, *Briefing for Cynical Commissioning Groups*, Health Emergency, http://www.healthemergency.org.uk/pdf/CynicalCommissioningGroups1.pdf 2014.

Instead, the special powers were used to fast track a deeply flawed plan, offering no facility for proper scrutiny of the TSA's actual proposals, which were then rubber-stamped by Jeremy Hunt with only minimal modification – more to the words than the substance of the plan. The plans to close and sell off two thirds of Lewisham Hospital were only eventually overturned through judicial review, which centred on a challenge to the powers of the TSA to act outside of the failing trust, not on the strength of the actual proposals themselves.[22] There was no chance to force the decision-makers to recognise the fictitious figures and projections on which they were based, or the wider threat to the viability of local services and impact on health care in south-east London. And without a massive protest on the streets and in the wider community around the threatened hospital there would have been no judicial review, and the flawed plan would have been implemented.

After even the TSA's powers proved inadequate to press through the closure of Lewisham Hospital, Jeremy Hunt resorted to more legislation to weaken the public voice. The 'hospital closure clause,' section 119 of the HSC Act, gives carte blanche for a future TSA to ride roughshod over local communities where they find it politically expedient to do so. Like the HSC Act, this was carried through parliament with LibDem support.[23]

The perceived need for this clause is testimony to the failure of the proponents of reconfiguration schemes to win any significant public support for their plans. However, it is probably of limited value. For any government to begin repeatedly to invoke Clause 119 and the Unsustainable Provider Regime would be a desperate undertaking, amounting to an admission of widespread failure of hospitals under their watch.

Proponents of the clause tried to reassure its many opponents by claiming that the process would be time limited, transparent and only used in specific circumstances – and be subject to public consultation, although experience of the existing TSA procedure shows this to be untrue. The passing of the clause suggests ministers and commissioners are prepared, where they feel they have no choice, to exploit this procedure to achieve reconfiguration not possible through standard planning procedures.

Even where no Trust Special Administrator was involved, consultation on reconfiguration was seriously limited in its scope, and CCGs were stubbornly resistant to taking any note of critical or opposing views – however well-founded. In west London this led to the railroading through of the inappropriately-named 'Shaping a Healthier Future', one of the biggest-ever closure plans – which called for the closure of four A&E units and two whole hospitals,* despite the absence of any serious plans (or resources) for adequate alternative services to be put in place before any were withdrawn. Whenever CCG chiefs were confronted by campaigners or the wider concerned public, they simply chose to ignore questions they could not answer, or refer people to the thousands of pages of confusingly written 'Business Case' documents – despite the fact that these inadequate plans and evidence-free policies were often the proof that the plan did not hang together.[24]

Ealing Council failed in its attempt to have these plans overturned on a judicial review (since in this case the extent of consultation and 'engagement' with the public was deemed by a judge to have been adequate), so once again the merits of the proposals, and viability of the resulting healthcare system were not even considered. However, Ealing Council did use its one last throw of the dice to invoke the residual powers of its Health Oversight and Scrutiny Committees, (powers left over from the original legislation that scrapped CHCs ten years earlier and not yet swept away by the Health and Social Care Act) to lodge a formal objection, forcing a decision on the closure plans from Jeremy Hunt as Secretary of State.[25]

Hunt responded by bringing in another relic of the mid-2000s, the Independent Reconfiguration Panel (IRP), to investigate. When the IRP reported, it did endorse the closure of the two smaller A&E units[26] – with, as we have since seen, disastrous consequences in terms of access to emergency services for patients in Hammersmith & Fulham and Brent, reducing parts of north-west London to one of the worst

* Hammersmith Hospital and Central Middlesex A&E departments, which have since closed, and virtually all acute and in-patient services as well as A&E at Charing Cross and Ealing Hospitals.

performances on A&E targets in the country. However the IRP was less than convinced by the robustness (or existence) of plans in 'Shaping a Healthier Future' to replace the services that would be lost with the closure of the two substantial hospitals, each with over 300 beds.[27] The commissioners and the two trusts involved were required to develop new plans – if need be going back to further consultation – and in the meantime to maintain existing services.

Straight after the IRP report the CCGs and Imperial Healthcare Trust which runs Charing Cross made clear their determination to forge ahead regardless, and plans have now been published by the Trust for the demolition of the majority of the Charing Cross site, and its sale to generate capital for investment in health care elsewhere.[28]

Local MP Andy Slaughter has summed up the way in which public voice has been excluded in this process:

There will be no public consultation on the plans for Charing Cross and St Mary's. Public information on the closure of Hammersmith and Central Middlesex A&E has not started, six weeks before closure, but £300,000 has been paid to PR consultants, including £55,000 to M&C Saatchi.

In February 2013 plans to sell the whole Charing Cross site save for a clinic on 3 per cent of the land were met with outrage and the local NHS promised to go away and think again. ... At the end of October Health Secretary Jeremy Hunt confirmed his wish to close Hammersmith A&E but said Charing Cross would 'continue to offer an A&E service'. ... Now we have the final proposals and they are worse than we were recently led to believe.

Charing Cross will close as a major hospital. It will be reduced to a primary care centre with some day surgery and treatment services. ... More than half the Charing Cross site will be sold, the existing hospital demolished and new building will provide less than a quarter of the current floor space. All consultant emergency services will close or go elsewhere. The present 360 inpatient beds will fall to just 24. The biggest betrayal is the loss of the A&E. Far from continuing 'to offer an A&E service' as Hunt promised, Imperial confirm that A&E will 'move out' of Charing Cross under their plans leaving 'an emergency service appropriate for a local hospital'. This means an urgent care centre staffed by GPs and nurses.[29]

So even where what remains of an appeals process appears to deliver a victory for the local community opposing a closure, there is no guarantee that the appeal rulings will be respected or upheld. The public voice is less powerful by far than the demands of the balance sheet and the drive for cash savings.

Since then it's been getting worse. At first, many of the reconfiguration plans had been drawn up by the primary care trusts and inherited by the CCGs. But now various CCGs have been seeking costly legal advice on how NOT to consult local people on substantial changes which they have themselves drawn up or taken responsibility for – such as the tendering of contracts, knowing that there will be no popular support for their proposals.

In Staffordshire, four of the county's CCGs, advised by the Macmillan cancer charity, are working together to put controversial contracts for the coordination of cancer services and end of life care (worth a combined £1.2 bn over ten years) out to tender. Huge public meetings and lobbies have repeatedly challenged the CCGs to publish their full proposals and name the companies that have expressed an interest. They have been met by a consistent refusal to share any real information – creating even more suspicion of the long-term implications of a process that could put a private company in charge of such a large budget for crucial services.

Suspicion is further raised by the publication via the EU of the initial invitation for tenders which makes clear that the only criterion for awarding the contract will be the 'most economically advantageous tender' – i.e. the cheapest, and the refusal to publish the Pre Qualification Questionnaire which 'will be used to determine the applicant's eligibility, economic and financial standing and technical ability'.

In Staffordshire and elsewhere, although CCGs themselves allegedly represent local GPs, the GPs are not really in charge at all. CCGs are all invariably run by a small handful of GPs, most often from the largest and most prosperous practices, who sit with other managers on the board. The CCG boards in turn are told what they can and can't do from above by bureaucrats from NHS England and its bureaucratic, secretive Local Area Teams (which also control local primary care services).

CCG boards seldom consult the wider local body of GPs, let alone allow them any kind of ballot or democratic vote on controversial policies. The one time this did happen, and a ballot was held among GPs in Surrey Downs CCG over a controversial plan threatening the future of the local Epsom Hospital and the relatively nearby St Helier in Carshalton – the majority delivered a resounding thumbs down to the proposals. The CCG was obliged to withdraw its support, and the entire 'Better Services Better Value' plan had to be abandoned.[30] Other CCGs have drawn the obvious lesson: don't ask GPs, or you may be forced to change course.

These unrepresentative bodies, now spurred on by the growing financial pressures of a frozen budget and constantly increasing pressures and demands on frontline services, are driving forward plans for reconfiguration of local NHS services. It seems the documents are largely based on blueprints and off-the-peg generic arguments and statistics supplied by NHS England, and often in open defiance of local public opinion.

Unlike PCTs and SHAs, CCGs have no responsibility to ensure the viability of local NHS providers or the local health economy – and some clearly feel free to take decisions which could seriously undermine local providers, despite long-term serious consequences for access to care for local populations.

There is no longer any wider system of regional overview to ensure the coherence of local plans. Local Area Teams of NHS England, which have now effectively replaced strategic health authorities, are not public bodies, appear to have no formal structure of meetings or public access to their discussions, publish no board papers, and avoid serious engagement or consultation with the local public at any level other than the highest level of abstraction.

There are also problems of reduced public voice in relation to the providers of health care. The Act requires all trusts to become foundation trusts, regardless of the fact that those which have not yet done so are almost all confronted by serious financial obstacles, and could well be driven in desperation to some of the cash-saving cuts in staffing that caused the massive crisis in Mid Staffordshire Hospitals Trust. Yet these changes in frontline care are not always visible in the high-level analysis presented in board meetings and published for local scrutiny.

Many foundation trusts still withhold publication of board

papers, and meet in secret with only minimal engagement with their own 'governors' rather than the wider local public even as their financial situation worsens. According to Monitor, more than half of the 164 foundations are now in deficit,[31] but the first local people are likely to hear about such problems is when substantial cutbacks or service changes are announced, and appear in the local news media.

Healthwatch

So what of the bodies that we might expect to represent the views of local people? Healthwatch (www.healthwatch. co.uk), which is organised at local and national level, was established under the HSC Act, subordinate to the Care Quality Commission. The new bodies were designed from the outset to be toothless, with a limited frame of reference, primarily offering advice, and with no independent role. They have been scarcely visible in many areas, in some cases openly arguing that their brief is not to campaign or speak up for local communities as the best of the old CHCs once did.

From a London perspective on what is clearly a national problem, the People's Inquiry into London's NHS, supported by Unite the union, concluded from the evidence heard that there seemed to be:

no real public awareness of, or confidence in the effective-ness of the new bodies established by the Health and Social Care Act to represent local views and give a limited degree of local accountability of NHS commissioners and providers.

Healthwatch, despite the efforts and good intentions of some working within the local groups, appears to be uneven and largely ineffective, with little if any public profile – and virtually no involvement in the issues that have galvanised the most active public interest in the last year. And in only one of our hearings (North Central London) was there a report indicating any impact or role for Health and Wellbeing Boards.[32]

The Inquiry also noted that in theory there should be a Healthwatch functioning in each London borough, but even where they do exist the local bodies lack both the legal powers of the old Community Health Councils and the expertise and links with the community that made the best CHCs a real force to be reckoned with. Even worse, while Healthwatch groups are supposed to be resourced by local authorities, a quarter of the funding that should have been funnelled to local Healthwatch groups from the Department of Health through their local councils had been siphoned off, and apparently used to pay other council bills instead – with no significant protest being raised.

In Bracknell, frustrated campaigners, seeing no sign at all of life in Healthwatch, have taken the initiative to set up their own, unofficial People's Healthwatch to keep a close eye on the local trusts and CCG and ensure that important issues are reported in local media. The first they heard from the official Healthwatch was a letter urging them not to choose a similar name, for fear of confusing people. The reply was that there could be no confusion, because no members of the public would ever have heard of the official Healthwatch!

The People's Inquiry concluded that Healthwatch in its current form is unlikely to deliver an effective voice for local communities, and recommended that they be wound up, with new bodies established that should be separated from the CQC and modelled on the old CHCs.

They should link up with local community organisations, pensioners groups and other community organisations, and be given the statutory powers to inspect hospital and community services, to object to changes which lack public acceptance, and to force a decision on contested changes from the Secretary of State.

The invisibility and impotence of Healthwatch is rivalled by many of the Health & Wellbeing Boards (HWBs), which were also established under the HSC Act. However HWBs are not NHS bodies, but controlled locally by councils with social service responsibilities. The unusual flexibility of the phrasing of the Act gives council extensive discretion on how public and outward-going the HWBs should be. There is the possibility to make them campaigning platforms, or a way to hold local health managers to account. But so far not one council has taken the chance to co-opt campaigners, community leaders and advocates of patient groups, and create HWBs as a vibrant, proactive public forum for scrutiny of local NHS commissioners or providers.

The London People's inquiry again recommended a substantial change, calling on councils to 'make under-achieving and narrow Health & Wellbeing Boards into genuine platforms for the planning and scrutiny of public health, health and social care in each borough'. It suggested that one way forward might even be to merge HWBs with Healthwatch,

to create a single, clear and authoritative, democratic voice for local people that will monitor and scrutinise local health and social care services and plans for future developments, but also champion patient complaints.

Of course, one other important player behind the scenes of CCGs, in addition to the control exercised by NHS England, is the shadowy network of 'commissioning support units', some of which are clearly steering the CCGs towards greater and wider moves to put services out to tender. These bodies too are beyond any public scrutiny or accountability, and it seems likely that many of them would be privatised if the Tories win the next election: they are all due to be put out to tender by 2016.

Conclusion

The whole sorry history of the erosion of the public voice since the late 1990s has been accelerated dramatically by the HSC Act and the cash pressures of the coalition's freeze on spending.

All this further exposes the cynical deception of Andrew Lansley's plagiarised promise that patients and public would be far more involved: 'nothing about me without me'. In fact almost every decision is now less likely than ever to be taken with any regard for the views and voice of patients, local communities or health professionals. The proliferation of commercial secrecy, from the very top right down to local commissioners and competing NHS trusts, means local people are even less likely to be aware of issues on which they might expect a say, and journalists find it harder than before to access information on controversial issues to inform their news audience.

The government's real agenda is opening up wider private sector involvement, replacing NHS providers with social enterprises and prioritising competition over cooperation, collaboration and quality of patient care. This is incompatible with democratic accountability and a strong independent voice for the public in influencing decisions. For people to take control, we need to dismantle the market and return the NHS to its founding values and purpose, allowing professionals to work together to address the health needs of local communities rather than tend the balance sheets of big business.

7

Myth: Our NHS reforms will make the NHS more transparent and accountable.

The NHS will become more transparent under proposals set out by the Health Secretary.[1]

Press release from Department of Health
and Andrew Lansley, October 2011

There was plenty of rhetoric about accountability and transparency in the period during the passage of the Health and Social Care Bill but an examination of the small print revealed that the reality would be different. There was an early indication of Lansley's real attitude to transparency when he refused to publish the risk register (which looked at the potential dangers if the Bill passed) despite having been ordered to do so by the Information Commissioner.

Clause 1 of the Bill ends the duty of the Secretary of State for health to 'secure or provide' a universal and comprehensive health service in England. This was a line in the sand for Lansley who was determined to make this change. The HSC Act has resulted in confused lines of accountability and a situation where a Secretary of State for health can criticise the NHS without offering solutions or acknowledging responsibility for problems arising from government policy.

Many features of the HSC Act conspire against transparency in the NHS. New bodies created by the Act do not have to meet in public or publish their minutes. There are different standards for the private sector delivering NHS care – they are protected by 'commercial confidentiality'. Information about their costs, profits and outcomes is unavailable and even parliamentary bodies struggle to find out the basic facts needed to assess their performance. Private companies are not subject to freedom of information requests. Despite promises to vet private companies bidding for NHS contracts there is no central register of 'Any Qualified Providers', nor any plan to establish one. Contrary to Lansley's promise the NHS is now considerably less transparent and accountable than it was before the HSC Act came into force.

* * *

The White Paper – a spurious promise of transparency

Within a few weeks of the 2010 election, in a Department of Health press release on the White Paper 'Equity and Excellence – Liberating the NHS',[2] Lansley made clear that in his new structure, the Secretary of State would no longer be in charge and therefore accountable for the NHS:

> But I want to be clear – while the NHS will no longer be accountable to ministers or the Department for its performance in these areas, it will be very much accountable to the patients and public it serves.[3]

Few people listening would have immediately drawn the conclusion from this that the very first clause of the HSC Bill (now the Act) would take the step of scrapping the Secretary of State's duty to provide universal and comprehensive health care, but of course it did.

A few days later, in a keynote policy speech to the NHS Confederation conference on 24 June 2010, Lansley claimed his White Paper, soon to be the Bill, represented a step towards transparency. He declared: 'I will set out what the Secretary of State is and is not responsible for, and where the Secretary of State is not responsible, I will set out who is.'[4]

Lansley's NHS Confederation speech also included a rousing commitment to 'democratic accountability'. He promised that:

> For the first time the voice of the public will be heard across commissioning, the public health service and social care. In these straitened financial times this accountability for how we use taxpayers' money is even more important.

Despite Lansley's fine phrases the 'voice of the public' has never been more marginalised than it has been since the HSC Act took effect (see Chapter 6). Not only did Lansley want to duck his own responsibility to steer the NHS, but he was also determined that the public would have no chance to hold commissioners or providers to account either.

Freedom of Information Act flouted

Of course Lansley was not the first to offer a false prospect of transparency while in reality reducing the level of public accountability for local services and NHS bodies. But by opening up the NHS to greater involvement with the private sector, the HSC Act also meant the further surrender of public sector values and potential for accountability, in favour of the secretive approach that is common in the private sector.

New Labour was obsessed with transforming the NHS from a public service into a purchaser of care from a competitive market for healthcare services. This and the resultant increasing use of private sector providers alienated many of its supporters in the years from 2000. New Labour ministers also shrouded whole new areas which once were in the public domain under a dense cloud of 'commercial confidentiality' – including competitive tenders, the contracts for Independent Sector Treatment Centres and outsourced diagnostic services, and the details of contracts for new hospitals built under PFI.

PFI contracts and the process through which the final deal was negotiated have always been and remain especially opaque. In some cases – even where local union reps have battled for years to invoke their rights to see the finished text of PFI contracts under the Freedom of Information Act – they have been handed only heavily redacted versions, often missing the very sections of most interest to them.[5]

While they were happy from time to time to take opportunist pot shots at secrecy under Labour, the Tories in government have been more than willing to behave in exactly the same way. The coalition government made clear from early on that they would pick and choose what information would be released not only to the wider public, but even to MPs deciding major policy changes.

The Risk Register
One of the early, unresolved battles around the HSC Bill concerned Lansley's dogged refusal to publish a 'risk register' compiled by Department of Health civil servants, exploring the potential dangers in the Bill and its implementation. Lansley defied not only the Labour opposition but also the Information Commissioner, who ruled that it was 'unjustified' to keep the register from MPs before they decided whether or not to support the huge Bill and its various clauses.[6] Lansley refused to budge, and the document was (and still is) withheld from everyone including MPs who, perhaps shockingly, voted by a majority that they were happy to decide on the Bill in ignorance of the warnings it contained.

In May 2012, just after the Bill completed its progress through Parliament, the Department of Health pronounced that the risk register would definitely not be published.[7] Instead a laundered 'review' of the Transition Risk Register was eventually published.[8] The register itself was eventually leaked to a few, including commentator Roy Lilley.[9]

Costly Powerpoint slides
One fascinating example of a complete lack of transparency was the major report from McKinsey that was commissioned by Labour ministers in 2009 (in the aftermath of the banking

crash), some elements of which leaked out to the health service trade press.[10] In it McKinsey consultants put forward ideas for steps to bridge the widening gap between an NHS budget that would no longer be growing in real terms and the rising demand for services.

In place of a proper, evidence-based and fully argued report, McKinsey produced a set of 124 largely unconnected Powerpoint slides (with no accompanying narrative or evaluation of the strengths and weaknesses of the various proposals). McKinsey argued that by 2015 the cumulative spending gap could be as high as £20bn – and then set out a series of increasingly speculative and largely unexplained ideas on how to generate up to £20bn of 'cost savings'.

The McKinsey document set out a wide range of proposals, but lacked any narrative explanation of how such measures were supposed to be implemented, or what any possible downsides and unintended consequences might be if they were. The evidence for most of their proposals was seriously deficient, or lacking altogether. But as news of the report leaked out in dribs and drabs, Labour ministers responded not only by denying that any of it was policy, and trying to distance themselves from having commissioned it – they refused point blank to publish it.

Lansley, then shadow health secretary, made great play of this in the run-up to the election, challenging and ridiculing Labour's secrecy. Indeed one of Lansley's first actions, once installed as Health Secretary in 2010, was to publish the McKinsey report, as he had promised.

However Lansley was also determined to enforce the £20bn savings target at the centre of the McKinsey plan. So denouncing and publishing the document turned out to be simply a prelude to Lansley effectively compelling almost all commissioners and many NHS trusts to adopt some of McKinsey's key proposals, and implement them in the quest for cost savings.

Since this one grand gesture of transparency (at the expense of the former government), the doors have swung completely shut once more. The drive towards greater secrecy has been resumed, taken to new levels by the fragmentation and attempts to foster competition set out in the HSC Act.

The McKinsey plans examined

Labour's suppression of the McKinsey proposals was most likely based on the document's potentially explosive content – not least the threat to over 100,000 NHS jobs – although it may also have been partly due to embarrassment at the poor quality of the report they had paid for, which was little more than a string of unsupported assertions.

Eerily foreshadowing the Five Year Forward View document produced in October 2014 by NHS England chief executive Simon Stevens,[11] the McKinsey suggestions began by insisting that heroic increases in productivity could be achieved – 15-22 per cent over three to five years, equivalent to £13-£20bn.*

But McKinsey went further: part of their £20bn target involved a 10 per cent reduction in staff – and a reduction in medical school training places to avert a surplus of doctors. Older GPs and community nursing staff would be offered early retirement. Staff who remained would be pressed to work more intensively, although how they could do that and maintain proper records and exchange information with

---

* The Stevens plan, welcomed by leaders of all three main parties, hopes to generate £22bn of efficiencies by 2021, with further savings to be made through a greater emphasis on prevention, which could lower demand for NHS treatment. Unlike Stevens, McKinsey did at least admit that this was unlikely to generate much in the first three to five years.

colleagues was not explained. The plans also demanded a concerted effort to push through hospital reconfigurations.

The drive for savings was broken down into eight main headings, including squeezing more 'productivity' out of acute hospitals (partly by reducing the tariff on which they would be paid for patient care) along with productivity savings from community and mental health services. There should be a programme of 'estates optimisation' – selling off 'spare' land and buildings.

Under 'optimising spending' came four pages of detailed suggestions on which treatments and operations the McKinsey team considered to offer 'no or limited clinical benefit', which many patients should therefore no longer be offered on the NHS – including some hip and knee replacements. Other types of treatment included on their list were tonsillectomy, back pain injections and fusion, grommets, hernia operations, varicose veins, minor skin surgery, cataract surgery and wisdom teeth extraction.

An expanded version of the document commissioned for NHS London included some added gems, such as the suggestion of cutting primary care consultation time by 33 per cent (from a target 12 minutes per patient to just 8) which McKinsey claimed could 'save' £570m.[12] While the authors may have accurately calculated this potential (notional) cash saving, they appear to have devoted no attention at all to a risk analysis of this policy, or considerations of quality from the patient and GP points of view. Obviously if cash savings are the sole objective, cutting GP consultation times by 60, 80 or even 100 per cent could increase the savings much further – although with more drastic and obvious impact on patient care.

It is easy to see why Labour might be especially keen to

keep these suggestions out of the public view, especially in the run-up to the forthcoming election. Andrew Lansley was equally determined, and much more successful, in the challenge of keeping his own plans – for a wholesale, top-down reorganisation of the NHS, and opening an ever-greater share of the NHS budget to potential private providers – out of sight until after the votes had been counted.

Retreating to arm's length

Clause 1 of the HSC Act ended the duty of the Secretary of State to secure or provide a universal and comprehensive health service in England. This responsibility was transferred to the body now known as NHS England. Lansley's successor as Health Secretary, Jeremy Hunt, has taken full advantage of the new scope this has given him.

Released from any formal responsibility Hunt has repeatedly used his position to criticise the NHS whenever things go wrong, while doing nothing to address the resource constraints or inefficiencies imposed upon it by his own government. In this way the HSC Act can be seen as a way of 'liberating' not the NHS but ministers – to attack it whenever they feel it politic to do so.

Hunt clearly feels free to point the finger of blame for any problems either at the local commissioners and providers of services, or at NHS England, the new national commissioning board which is now theoretically responsible for commissioning – while the responsibility for frontline services remains firmly on the local NHS trust or Foundation Trust.

Lib Dem minister Norman Lamb has taken similar advant-age of the separation of the NHS from parliamentary control, washing his hands of any responsibility for NHS England's decision to impose bigger cuts on mental health budgets than on acute hospitals.

Speaking to the NHS Confederation's Mental Health Network,[13] Lamb criticised NHSE's decision to impose a tariff reduction of 1.8 per cent in mental health contracts, compared with 1.5 per cent in acute care. He told delegates the decision was 'flawed, not based on evidence and cannot be defended'. But then he dumped the problem straight back onto the mental health trusts, saying they should 'fight' with their commissioners over their contracts: 'Do not accept a proposed settlement which results in mental health losing out.'

Since his Tory bosses have (with LibDem support) forced through legislation that puts all of the financial control in the hands of commissioners, and all of the problems in the court of the provider trusts, this is a cynical, hypocritical evasion.

However, Lamb's outburst did at least confirm that the bold proposals of the Department of Health's 'Closing the Gap' report,[14] launched by Lamb and Nick Clegg in January 2014 with the declared aim of working towards 'parity of esteem' between mental and physical health care, were not worth the paper they are written on. Having set up a dysfunctional system, Lib Dem ministers and Tories alike intend to stand back and blame the NHS as things go horribly wrong.

Now the Secretary of State is no longer responsible, in theory accountability for our health services runs through a variety of bureaucratic bodies. The Act established a new NHS Commissioning Board, now known as NHS England, which is responsible overall for the commissioning of primary care and specialist services, and for vetting the constitutions, setting the budgets and monitoring the decisions of all 211 local commissioners (Clinical Commissioning Groups).

The new regulator of the NHS is an expanded version of Monitor, which was set up by Labour in 2004 to regulate foundation trust hospitals. The regulator of quality and patient safety is the Care Quality Commission. On top of this there is the least well-known regulator of all, the Medicines and Healthcare products Regulatory Agency (MHRA) whose impotence was clearly demonstrated during the PIP breast implants scandal (see Chapter 8). However not one of these bodies, which are supposed to be the vehicle for accountability and transparency, is either accountable or transparent.

Not so open – NHS England

NHS England makes a great show of holding its board meetings not only in public but streamed on the Internet, but the agendas make clear that the meetings are dealing with only a small part of the business that passes through NHS England.

On a day-to-day basis much of the activity flows instead through NHS England's network of Local Area Teams (LATs). These are the even more bureaucratic and secretive equivalent of the old strategic health authorities (SHAs). However, unlike the old SHAs, the LATs appear to have no formal structure of meetings, and offer no public access to board meetings or to board papers. They are 'accountable' only vertically upwards to NHS England and not at all downwards to the towns, cities and communities whose health services are subject to their decisions.

They may be obscure bodies to the public and health workers, but the LATs exercise real power over local services, shaping NHS England decisions over allocations to primary care and specialist services. Both of these face considerable problems.

After years of steadily declining allocations of NHS resources to primary care,[15] planned revisions to the funding for GP services in deprived areas threatened to make significant numbers of GP practices unsustainable, effectively forcing their closure, until a last-minute change of policy.[16] GPs, led by the Royal College of General Practitioners, are campaigning for an increased share of the NHS budget to be allocated to primary care, which, according to NHS England[17] and the Royal College of General Practitioners,[18] handles around 90 per cent of all daily encounters with patients – for less than 9 per cent of the funding.

Meanwhile there have been continuing arguments over NHS England's inept commissioning of mental health services, which led to them attempting to impose a tariff for secure forensic services which favoured poor quality private services over top quality and effective NHS care.[19] While a makeshift formula has so far been able to protect the NHS trusts that would have lost out on this formula, problems of desperate shortages of specialist inpatient services for Child and Adolescent Mental Health Services (CAMHS) have continued unabated, with some children transported up to 275 miles across the country in search of a bed. There are also serious shortages of appropriately-trained CAMHS staff, community based services, and intensive outreach teams, resulting in delays in discharging those patients who have managed to access services.[20]

As this chapter is completed comes news that in another abrupt retreat NHS England has been forced to abandon its silly plan to incentivise GPs to diagnose dementia in older patients with a 'bounty' of £50 for each diagnosis. The plan has been 'ended before it even began'.[21]

NHS England's lack of local accountability and transparency, and the difficulty local communities and health professionals have in engaging with its far from accessible LATs have compounded these problems. They leave plenty of scope for further policy blunders and omissions in future, as the board attempts to rein in overspending of almost £400m in 2013-14.[22]

Monitor – a confused watchdog

Similar problems of accountability and transparency apply to the workings of Monitor, which since the HSC Act is the overall regulator of the NHS, setting prices for NHS-funded care and compiling a register of 147 foundation trusts and 96 private providers who are licensed to deliver NHS-funded treatment.

The HSC Act also gave Monitor a contradictory brief, making it responsible both for ensuring 'integration' of services *and* for preventing 'anti-competitive' behaviour (i.e. promoting competition). Monitor has been criticised for using its powers to license Foundation Trusts as a way to scale back hospital and community services in England. This threatens to reduce NHS-funded care after 2016 (when new regulations come into force) to a 'basic package of services equivalent to those that must be provided in the event of foundation trust failure'.[23]

Meanwhile the Commons Public Accounts Committee has expressed different concerns over Monitor and its ability to cope with its expanded brief. It points out that Monitor is hampered by a lack of clinical expertise and frontline NHS management experience. Just 21 of its 337 staff have an NHS operational background, and only seven are clinicians, meaning that 92 per cent of Monitor's staff have no appropriate background for the role they are supposed to play. By contrast no fewer than thirty people are employed on PR spin in Monitor's huge department of 'strategic communications'.[24]

Almost 20 per cent of Monitor's £45m budget is spent hiring external management consultants to fill gaps in expertise and make up the numbers. Even with these staff, who do not assist in the development of in-house knowledge, Monitor is still 25 per cent short of the 450 staff it estimates are needed to fulfil its obligations properly. It is not clear who is accountable for regulating and scrutinising the work of this regulator.

Not so transparent foundations

One of the least transparent parts of the NHS has been the foundation trusts, many of which have eagerly exploited the 'freedom' to hold their regular meetings in secret and publish no board papers. The HSC Act offers them even more dubious 'freedoms', allowing them to raise up to half of their income from delivering private medicine to paying patients, or contracts with the private sector. The public have had no opportunity to express their views on these changes let alone vote on them; in fact most of the MPs nodding through the Bill that encouraged NHS hospitals to open more private beds and private clinics clearly had no idea what they were supporting.

Although the Act makes a token concession to some level of accountability by requiring a foundation trust to get support from its Board of Governors for such a policy, it is already clear that many foundations have forged ahead regardless, and expanded their private work substantially since the HSC Act became law.

Even if the governors were involved in some tokenistic level of discussion it is clear that these changes are taking place with no engagement or transparency as far as the local public are concerned. By lifting restrictions on how much private money can be made in this way ordinary NHS patients cease to be the priority of some foundation trust managements, and become virtual second-class citizens compared with those with money to pay for their treatment.

Who is 'qualified'?

The HSC Act has put the entire NHS at arm's length from any democratic accountability, while at the same time opening the door for a growing range of services to be further distanced through contracts with 'any qualified provider'.

Among Monitor's obligations is the requirement to vet the private companies ('qualified providers') bidding for NHS contracts.* The Department of Health's Operational Guidance to the NHS on 'Extending Patient Choice of Provider', published back in 2011 assured us that the 'key principles' of Any Qualified provider (AQP) were that: 'Providers qualify and register to provide services via an assurance process that tests providers' fitness to offer NHS-funded services ... Competition is based on quality, not price.'[25]

However this is simply not happening. Shockingly neither Monitor nor the CQC currently holds or publishes any register of qualified providers. Monitor does not even bother to licence any organisation that has contracts with the NHS of less than £10m per year – thus excusing the vast majority of smaller 'alternative' providers and non-profit businesses from seeking any licence.

A call to Monitor by this author has confirmed that they have no register of AQP companies and organisations, nor

---

* The contracts themselves were also supposed to be regulated and scrutinised by the other main 'arm's length' regulatory body, the Care Quality Commission.

any plans to establish one. Indeed they would 'love to know where there is a list'. Nor, it seems, is NHS England doing the job; they refer inquiries on to the Department of Health. The Department in turn appears to have decided to abandon its role in checking the credentials of would be private providers. It ceased to provide central support on this for commissioners as of 14 March 2014: 'From 2014/15 onwards, qualification of providers will be entirely for commissioners to take forward with support from Commissioning Support Services, as required.'[26]

In the spring of 2014, the online 'AQP Resource Centre' was closed down as part of the Supply2Health website, which is also now defunct. Yet another responsibility has in this way been dumped back onto the local level by those supposed to be scrutinising and regulating NHS services. This opens a real possibility of a postcode lottery in which certain companies will be accepted as 'qualified' by some CCGs, but not by others, and where lessons learned in one location have no means of transmission to other potential commissioners. The system now makes it difficult even to develop the equivalent of the 'Trip Advisor' website which allows consumers (satisfied or not) to feed back on their experience of hotels, resorts and restaurants.

This is a long way from transparency, and leaves huge scope for companies delivering poor and inadequate care to secure and retain 'qualified' status. Unlike NHS trusts, private companies delivering NHS clinical and other services are not subject to the Freedom of Information Act, allowing them to hide a multitude of potential sins and omissions.

Meanwhile there are question marks over the definition of 'qualified' – and whether the qualifications are appropriate. In the spring of 2013, as Clinical Commissioning Groups began to function in earnest, a search through the online lists of 'any qualified providers' revealed that a company known as 'Minor Ops Ltd' had been deemed qualified to deliver Adult Podiatry services in Darlington and County Durham. The company was given the contract as a parting shot by the Primary Care Trust.[27] On closer inspection, four of the seven providers working under the label of 'Minor Ops Ltd' turn out to be optometrists or opticians – not the kind of specialists people with foot problems would normally expect to consult. The same company also operates on eyelids!

When is 'NHS' not really NHS?

Exploiting the freedoms of the market system that has been put in place, many profit-seeking private companies increasingly treat NHS patients in premises bearing the NHS logo, leaving them confused as to who is actually providing the care even if the NHS is footing the bill. Once again transparency is almost impossible when such details are obscured from public view. This can also mean that when a private provider delivers an inferior or unsafe service under the NHS logo, the NHS takes the blame.

Confidence in Monitor's scrutiny of contracts and contractors is not enhanced by the fact that since September 2013 it has relied on contracts with ten management and accounting firms to help develop plans for failing foundation trusts, and its resulting bill for consultancy fees has soared to more than six times the amount it was spending before the Act was passed.

Six big firms* picked up work worth between £1.7m and £11.3m from Monitor in 2013-2014, adding up to £28.3m that

* In ascending order of consultancy fees: FTI consulting, Deloitte, KPMG, McKinsey, PricewaterhouseCoopers, and Ernst & Young.

year. These include the four accountancy firms criticised by Margaret Hodge, chair of the Commons Public Accounts Committee, for providing advice to government on how to design tax laws, while simultaneously advising rich corporate clients on how to evade them.[28]

It should be no surprise that Monitor is so closely tied to the management consultancy firms. Its chief executive David Bennett (who for years was also chair), was formerly a senior partner at McKinsey, and half a dozen of Monitor's directors and senior managers have links to management consultancy and city law firms.[29] Its interim chair until the end of 2014 was Baroness Hanham, a senior Tory and former leader of the London Borough of Kensington & Chelsea.

Careless Quality Commission

Another prominent Tory political appointee chairs the Care Quality Commission (CQC), which is the body responsible for checking whether hospitals, care homes, GPs, dentists and domiciliary services are meeting national standards. David Prior was formerly a Tory MP and deputy chairman of the Conservative Party.

The CQC inspects services and publishes its findings, 'helping people to make choices about the care they receive' and as such its role has been subject to frequent, withering attacks from commentator Roy Lilley on his website www.nhsmanagers.net. Lilley points out that the arrival of coachloads of CQC inspectors seeking to find fault (on what are often relatively marginal criteria and formal 'checklists') – while offering no solutions – is not the way to improve performance or morale. He refers to US systems expert Edwards Deming: 'We know Deming is right about inspection; Cease dependence on inspection to achieve quality. Eliminate the need for massive inspection by building quality into the product in the first place.'[30]

David Prior demonstrated scant faith in the health service his organisation is supposed to inspect (and incurred the wrath of the *Daily Mail*) by going private for a hip operation early in 2014, 'bypassing NHS waiting times – which are the longest they have been for three years'.[31] In March 2014, Prior gave a speech in which he backed the idea of bringing in 'successful operators of foreign hospital chains' to turn around what he predicted could be up to thirty failing NHS organisations.[32] The clear implication that this could open up the NHS to private hospital chains and multinationals was not lost on campaigners.

The CQC is still rebuilding its tattered reputation, having been caught in a protracted row over accountability for the delays in identifying poor quality care at Mid Staffordshire Hospitals Trust in 2006-7. Now it has also been criticised for lacking the leadership, resources and skills to check on the quality of care in hospitals and thousands of privately-run care homes, let alone the work of 40,000 GPs.

Ineffectual

The least well-known regulator, the Medicines and Health-care products Regulatory Agency (MHRA), was shown in the arguments over poor quality breast implants supplied by a French company to be largely ineffectual, and operating under the thumb of EU and European governments.

In 2012 an editorial in the *Lancet* accused the MHRA of having been aware of the risks of serious device failures for some time, and described the PIP implant scandal as 'an inevitable result of MHRA's paralysis and inability to correct the failings of a severely flawed system'. It claimed the MHRA operated under the principle of 'do nothing until something goes wrong'.[33]

Trade treaties and competition law

Bad as they may be, all of these organisations are models of transparency and accountability compared with what could be unleashed on the NHS by the full weight of EU competition law, asserting the 'right to provide' for private sector companies trying to muscle in on large, attractive public sector budgets, and potentially exploiting the new competitive market created by the HSC Act.

On top of this comes the threat that, urged on by the Cameron government, the EU will sign up for the controversial Transatlantic Trade and Investment Partnership (TTIP) which – under the spurious banner of 'free trade' – seeks to stack the odds overwhelmingly on the side of US multinationals seeking rich pickings from Europe's public sector.[34] This would open up the possibility of legal challenges by corporations being decided in special secret courts – as part of an apparatus that subordinates matters such as patient care, quality of services and collaboration to advance medical knowledge to the great god of 'competition'.[35]

TTIP is unlikely to be the final effort to prise open public sector budgets for a frustrated private health sector that has shown itself unable to develop any genuine 'market' without the help of political patronage, tax breaks, concessions and skewed legal systems. Each additional treaty is therefore likely to further override and obstruct any transparency or accountability.

Existing competition laws, the problems of replacing a failed provider once the NHS services have been privatised – and the fear of legal challenge – are already making it difficult for timid NHS commissioners to get rid of failing private sector providers.[36] All this is set to get worse if these new treaties are signed and more contracts are awarded to private providers under the HSC Act section 75.

As Bones might have said to Captain Kirk on the Starship *Enterprise*, as a one-time public service drifted off the starboard bow, visibly transforming into a competitive market, 'It's transparency Jim, but not as we know it'.

ncreasingly a myth as Chapter 3 has demonstrated), and
ality of providers' (weasel words for private companies)
ow discredited, but still the politicians press on. Much
e move towards privatisation of the NHS has taken place
ealth and behind closed doors but when called upon to
nd it the cheerleaders use the free market argument –
NHS will benefit from more private sector involvement
use commercial companies will do things more cost-
ctively and more efficiently than the public sector, and
oring innovation to the service.

ere's the evidence?

ence of the inherent superiority of the private sector in
ering public services is non-existent, notwithstanding
claims of those who advocate outsourcing the NHS.
ed the available evidence points to quite the reverse.
need only to look at the US which has long provided a
warning about the perils of outsourcing health care.
icians dismiss comparisons with the US and reassure us
we are not going down 'the American route', but in fact
nificant percentage of US health care is publicly funded
privately delivered and thus forms a useful indication of
this market-based system works. For example, the US
em of Medicare (the social insurance programme for
rly people, with a budget twice that of the entire NHS) is
d on the same combination of public funding and private
very that is being forced on the NHS.
avid Woolhandler and Steffie Himmelstein, two Harvard
essors, in a seminal paper from 2007[6] asked whether
UK was right to adopt a market model for improving
ealth services. Their answer was an unequivocal and
ence-based 'No', and concluded with a warning to the

8

Myth: The private sector is more efficient and cost-effective than the public sector.

*[P]ush ahead with a steady increase in private provision to
raise standards and encourage better value for money through
the trial and error of the marketplace.*[1]

David Green, *Daily Telegraph*, 11 May 2011

… privatise and efficiency will almost automatically increase.[2]

Oliver Letwin, *Privatising the World*

There is no evidence that the private sector is cheaper or
more cost effective when it delivers public health care. The
only evidence available shows the reverse: that costs go up
and the quality of the service goes down.

The Health and Social Care Act moves us towards an
NHS where care is still publicly funded but is increasingly
outsourced to the private sector. The US system of Medicare
runs along the same lines as those being forced on the NHS,
i.e. publicly funded but privately delivered. A 2007 paper in
the *British Medical Journal* warned the UK not to follow the
same route.

There are many well documented problems that arise
when health care is outsourced to the private sector, and we
are already seeing all of these affecting the NHS since the
passage of the HSC Act.

- Worse outcomes for patients.
- Cherry picking patients to increase profits.
- Greatly increased administration costs arising from the marketisation of the NHS.
- Destabilisation of the public service.
- Antisocial behaviour by the private sector.
- Loss of accountability and transparency.

Outsourcing NHS care involves running the service as a market and the associated costs are high. It is imperative to avoid waste at a time of 'austerity', which makes it even more surprising that the coalition has chosen to waste £5-10bn a year of scarce NHS resources on marketising the English NHS.

A blind faith in the power of the market to work its wonders is no substitute for evidence of benefit and there is none. Indeed the reverse is the case – privatisation is inefficient and outsourcing public services represents the worst type of mixed economy – private companies take the profits while society underwrites the risks.

* * *

*Corporations have been enthroned and an e
in high places will follow.*[3]

A

*Why should the private sector be any better
services than the NHS? The simple answer is*

One of the great strengths of the NHS is th
recently it has been largely publicly delive
ance of public *delivery* cannot be overstate
been and still is delivered by NHS staff in
and by GPs who have long been regarde
part of the NHS. This means that taxpaye
back into the public purse to be spent on
than being diverted to shareholders' profit
Patients benefit from collaboration rather
between different parts of the NHS, and ar
faced with a fragmented service and a po
what is available. Staff throughout the NH
pay and conditions. The public sector eth
and appreciated by patients, most of who
well what happens when public services su
outsourced or simply privatised. All the e
that the NHS is a good example of a su
effective public service (see Chapter 2).

Nevertheless all major political parties,
years, have to a greater or lesser degree p
the direction of the private sector. The story
governments have introduced the priva
NHS through the back door has been we
The language is now becoming stale witl
like 'patient choice' (the Trojan horse for

UK to quarantine rather than replicate the US experience with Medicare. The paper is essential reading for those who want the evidence about outsourcing national health care, and much of it looks depressingly familiar. It warned that when private companies took over the delivery of public health care it was followed by worse outcomes for patients, cherry picking of profitable patients, soaring administration costs, public money diverted to profits, fraud on an industrial scale, kickbacks for doctors, the abandoning of unprofitable contracts, and eventual government bale-outs for private companies who couldn't make a profit despite employing all of these tactics.

But such hard facts have never been allowed to dent ideological commitment to the private sector and to the market. The enthusiasts seem to think that mindless repetition will triumph – that if they repeat the mantra about private sector efficiency and cost-effectiveness often enough it will be true or at least that we the public will believe it to be true. So it is vital to collect and lay out the evidence against private involvement in the delivery of health care.

However this is surprisingly difficult. Politicians constantly call for vigilance and transparency in public services but have double standards when it comes to the private sector. Private companies providing NHS care are not expected to meet the same standards of transparency as the publicly delivered NHS; for instance they are not subject to Freedom of Information requests, and as a result much about them is shrouded in secrecy. Their costs, profits and most importantly their outcomes are largely unknown, withheld from those who are paying for and using the self-same services. 'Commercial confidentiality' is paramount and overrules patients' and taxpayers' interests. Margaret Hodge, chair of the Public

Accounts committee, once famously complained that even her committee could not get behind the wall of secrecy erected by the commercial sector. It is therefore easy for the peddlers of the market to continue to claim its benefits while having conveniently few facts to back up their claims.*

In the absence of evidence we are left with anecdote and there is no shortage of that. And while Woolhandler's and Himmelstein's warnings to the UK about the dangers of a marketised health system were not comprehensive they serve as a good place to start.

Worse outcomes for patients

The 2007 paper reported higher death rates in the US in privately-run hospitals and renal dialysis centres than in not-for-profit ones. Concerns about outcomes for NHS patients treated in the private sector have been around for years but, in the absence of any government data, have been difficult to prove. What we do know comes largely from anecdotal evidence and from research conducted by clinicians and campaigners.

In 2009 hard evidence appeared when the *Journal of Bone and Joint Surgery* published a paper[7] which reported a much higher than expected rate of problems following hip replacements carried out on NHS patients in a privately run Independent Sector Treatment Centre (ISTC). The authors blamed poor technique, but this was not their only worry. The problems were only detected because of concerns raised by the local NHS about the surgical results at the ISTC, and the patients had then to be sorted out by the NHS. The authors drew attention not only to the poor outcomes for patients but also warned that detecting the problems and dealing with

---

* See Chapter 7 for more detail on transparency.

them had impacted significantly on the work of their NHS unit.

The paper concluded by asking that in future

> Contracts should not be renewed (for ISTCs) and new contracts should not be signed until a proper independent evaluation has been published assessing referrals, actual treatments carried out and payments made for work done along with value for money analysis. Full contract details and costs must be placed in the public domain for this assessment to take place.

Needless to say the paper received little national coverage and their recommendations fell on deaf ears. Commercial confidentiality continues to trump every other interest including that of the patients. An article in *Hospital Doctor*[8] summarised the known problems with ISTCs and concluded 'if ISTCs are providing treatment at higher costs than the mainstream NHS, with poorer outcomes, why are we sending our patients to them?' Why indeed.

In September 2013 the BBC reported that a privately-run ISTC had been taken back under NHS control after the unexpected deaths of three patients after routine surgery for joint conditions.[9] The Surgicentre (run by Clinicenta, a subsidiary of the giant construction and facilities company Carrillion) provided routine operations for NHS patient from the nearby Lister hospital. In 2012 the Care Quality Commission (CQC) failed it in four out of five areas and local GPs had 'decided to adopt a policy of dissuading their patients from being treated by the private care provider'.

The deaths were described as 'unfortunate' by the Clinicenta clinical director and as 'serious incidents' by the local NHS, and they contributed to the '21 serious incidents of both a clinical and patient information governance nature' since the clinic had opened in 2011.[10] They also followed an investigation at the centre earlier in the same year after six patients suffered 'irreversible sight loss', due to 'a lack of follow up care after treatment'.[11] GPs were warned that they should not 'refer patients to a service for which they have ... genuine concerns that the quality is substandard'.[12]

A local Tory MP, Stephen McPartland, was appropriately outraged, calling for the private clinic to be closed. Christine McAnea of Unison commented that the government's drive to privatisation was putting patients at clinical risk in a fragmented health service and that while politicians talked about patient choice, patients could not have known about the risks when they chose the privately-run Surgicentre for their NHS operation. 'These companies see the HSCA as a big opportunity to increase their business, but safeguarding patients has to be the number one priority.'[13]

In June 2014 the Bureau of Investigative Journalism broke a story about a private company, Healthcare at Home (or not, as the case may be), who were contracted to deliver medicines to seriously ill patients in their own homes.[14] The Bureau revealed that due to failures in the service patients had been left waiting for vital prescriptions, some of which had not arrived in time. Affected patients had had to fight to get through on the company's busy phone lines and patients were left 'confused and uncertain about when and whether their medication would arrive'.

Problems had arisen because distribution had been subcontracted out, and because extra patients had been taken on when another company, Medco Health Solutions, withdrew from the market only three years after entering it.

Patient groups described the failures as 'unacceptable and unsafe' and 'appalling' and had spent 'hours every week' sorting out problems. Several hospitals stopped using the service or fined them for failed deliveries. In March 2014 the company said it was no longer accepting new 'high risk' patients.

Perhaps the most alarming part of the story is reserved for the end. The Bureau reported that despite what had happened the Department of Health had asked the company to re-tender to be part of a panel of firms providing drug delivery services to the NHS. The Haemophilia Society, some of whose patients had been affected by the firm's failures, was involved in the decision making process. Their Chief executive, Liz Carroll, complained that they were not allowed to take account of Healthcare at Home's past performance when deciding on whether they should be on the new panel.

We have been advised that when making a decision on which firms should be included in the panel we can only consider the content of the bids. We are not allowed to take the company's past performance into consideration. We have asked for that to be changed. As a patient organisation we cannot just forget the experience of our members.

Not only were no lessons learned, they were apparently *wilfully ignored*. The implication is that when the private sector is involved it is acceptable to overlook the track record and concentrate on the promises, the marketing strategy of snake oil salesmen through the ages.

In August 2014 the Centre for Health and the Public Interest (CHPI), a progressive think tank, published a report about patient safety in private hospitals. It noted that over 800 patients had died unexpectedly in private hospitals in England during the previous four years. It surmised that this might in part be due to lack of appropriate staff, equipment and facilities. Three of their main findings are of major concern and are worth quoting in full:

- The majority of private hospitals have no intensive care beds, some have no dedicated resuscitation teams, and surgeons and anaesthetists usually work in isolation – without assistant surgeons and anaesthetists in training present.
- Although the private hospital sector now gets over a quarter of its income from treating NHS-funded patients, there is significantly less information available to patients about the performance of private hospitals than about the NHS.
- It is not possible to establish whether all private hospitals providing NHS care are fulfilling their legal obligation to publish Quality Accounts letting the public know how they are performing ....

The report also confirmed another problem which has long been known about but never officially recognised: that the private sector uses the NHS as a safety net or – rather more unceremoniously – a dumping ground when it runs into trouble. The report highlighted that:

- thousands of people are regularly transferred to NHS hospitals following treatment in private hospitals, with over 2,600 emergency NHS admissions from the private sector in 2012-13.[15]

In summary, while private hospitals are increasingly turning to the NHS for their income (see Chapter 9) they may not always be equipped to deal with the problems that arise, which they may then transfer back to the NHS. Information which would allow patients to exercise 'choice', in particular about private hospital performance, is in short supply. We don't have the government to thank for this important information, crucial to the interests of taxpayers, patients and voters, but a progressive think tank (CHPI) which went to the trouble to do the unfunded and uninvited research.

It is worth noting in passing that the average private hospital has fifty beds. As they don't deal with emergencies they tend to bring surgical staff in on a sessional basis and they don't have junior staff resident as they don't train doctors. This may be fine for routine work but not when emergencies arise, hence their use of the NHS as a backstop.

The buck stops where exactly?

There is still an alarming lack of clarity about who is liable when things go wrong for NHS patients being treated in private facilities. In August 2014 the *BMJ* reported that Musgrove Park, an NHS hospital, had terminated a contract with a private provider, Vanguard, after only four days when half of the sixty patients who had undergone cataract operations were found to have experienced complications.[16] One patient lost his sight and was told he would need a corneal transplant. There was immediate confusion about where liability lay and the patients' solicitor Laurence Vick referred to the 'uneasy relationship' between the NHS and the private sector. 'Private providers must agree to an immediate joint investigation with the NHS of problems on contracts, in place of the current fragmented approach.' It was also not clear whether the NHS hospital could recoup its losses after ending the contract. It was left to Vick to comment that 'from the taxpayer's point of view it would be totally unreasonable for Vanguard to walk away from this scandal with only their reputation, and not their investment, damaged'.[17]

In September 2014 *The Guardian* reported that Musgrove Park had carried out its own investigation (more NHS money spent on sorting out problems with the private sector) but was reluctantly refusing to publish it after lawyers had advised that 'individuals and parties might sue for defamation'.[18] It looked very much as though the NHS was afraid of publishing the truth about what had happened: an unacceptable outcome for the patients concerned. Vick commented:

> We have been waiting for this investigation for five months, and it is imperative that it is released to the public. The fear is that, when the private sector is involved, there can be absence of transparency that has become a reassuring feature of the NHS. There is concern as to whether the NHS should outsource to a private health sector that is still inadequately regulated. Private companies have a duty to shareholders as well as patients.

Shortly thereafter the report was leaked and confirmed many of the problems dogging outsourced contracts. Vanguard had undertaken to perform twenty operations a day, six more than the hospital's own doctors would do in a day. The firm had subcontracted the supply of surgeons and equipment to another company which had further subcontracted the supply of some equipment. This combination had not been tried before and training was still going on when the first patients arrived at the mobile operating theatre.[19] The refusal to publish the report even after it was leaked made a mockery of the government's promise of transparency after the Mid Staffs scandal.

It is not possible in a book of this scope to give a comprehensive list of all the evidence that has emerged about poor outcomes for NHS patients at the hands of the private sector and the reader is referred to the reading list at the end of the book for a guide to further sources. It is important to note that the failures have often had to be uncovered by investigative journalists, patient groups, NHS campaigners and progressive think tanks, and not by the government or the Department of Health. It suggests that the government is either having difficulty in monitoring the increasingly privatised and fragmented NHS, or that, for ideological reasons, it has double standards when it comes to the private sector, or more likely both.

The private sector must be treated in the same way as the NHS in all regards, including publishing its outcomes and being held to public account for its failures, but that is still not the case. Until that happens we are left guessing as to whether the horror stories that surface give us the whole picture or are just the tip of an iceberg that the government, despite their calls for openness and transparency, would rather keep submerged.

Fraud and corruption

A 2014 *BMJ* editorial estimated that 'between 10% and 25% of global spend on public procurement of health is lost through corruption' and identified it as 'one of the biggest open sores in medicine'.[20] The US was singled out as having lost between $82 and $272bn to medical embezzlement in just one year (2011), and as an 2014 *Economist* article (The $272 billon swindle) amply demonstrated, healthcare fraud in the US is big business.[21]

The potential for fraud and corruption in the NHS has traditionally been low. The conditions in which they flourish – lack of accountability and external oversight, doctors working in private systems who are incentivised to generate income by over investigation and overtreatment of patients, and a culture that accepts corruption – are lacking. But some of that is set to change after the HSC Act.

A marketised NHS means there are escalating numbers of financial transactions to monitor, but adequate oversight of the increasingly fragmented system is nigh on impossible, and will remain so as more 'qualified providers' come onto the scene. In addition there was previously little or no financial incentive for NHS doctors to refer patients for unnecessary investigations and treatments, a potent source of fraud and waste in the US. But as a result of the HSC Act GPs control much of the budget and, as a signifiant number of GPs on Clinical Commissioning Groups (CCGs) have financial interests in healthcare providers, concerns about financial conflicts of interest are bound to increase.

In 2013 the *BMJ* used Freedom of Information requests and CCG websites to discover that more than a third of GPs on CCGs had 'a conflict of interest due to directorships or shares held in private companies'. The *BMJ* editor Fiona Godlee commented:

> Some of these conflicts of interest are too great to be 'managed'. We think those GPs who have positions at executive board level in private provider companies need to choose between their competing interests and, if need be, step down from the commissioning boards.[22]

But later that year *Pulse* magazine reported that one in five GPs sitting on CCGs had a financial stake in a private company which was currently providing services *to their own CCG*.[23]

When, in 2014, the West Sussex CCG awarded a £235m contract for musculoskeletal (MSK) services to BUPA it was reported that only seven out of a possible 21 people responsible for the decision were actually able to vote on it, as the others all had financial conflicts of interest. The process was halted after local protests and the discovery that the CCG had done little to determine how their decision would impact on local hospitals.

West Sussex Hospitals NHS Trust, who had unsuccessfully bid for the contract, pointed out the obvious problems arising from the decision. The staff working in the trust MSK service were also responsible for emergency trauma care in their A&E department, so moving the MSK contract out of the trust would threaten their ability to staff the emergency services. Dr Armstrong, the chief officer of the CCG, said there was no intention to destabilise local A&E and trauma services, although she didn't explain how these would be maintained with the profitable part of the service contracted out. At the time of writing the decision is still under review.[24]

The story illustrates the problems facing CCGs and raises important concerns. Even if those with conflicts of interest leave the room for the vote it is difficult to think that they will not influence the decision made by a small group of their colleagues who remain behind.

In Bedfordshire they didn't even bother to vote. The CCG awarded a five year £120m contract for MSK services to a consortium led by Circle which included a company (Horizon Health Choices) whose website announces that it is owned by 25 of the 55 GPs practices in Bedfordshire. When challenged on the propriety of GPs on the CCG board voting on this the response was that no vote was taken since the policy went through by consensus. This effectively ignored the massive potential conflict of interest in agreeing a decision that would benefit colleagues, if not the board members themselves.

It eventually emerged that with the chutzpah characteristic of the private sector Circle intended to subcontract part of the work back to Bedford Hospital, the local NHS trust. The trust refused to become a subcontractor, preferring to compete with them, having seen a 30 per cent drop in its MSK referrals after Circle won the contract.[25]

This does not mean decisions made by CCGs are likely to be fraudulent, but that for the first time a culture has been created in which fraud and corruption are possible. Until now patients have trusted their GP's advice to be untainted by suspicions of financial gain. Once GPs are known to have financial interests in local health providers from whom they are purchasing services then patients will inevitably be concerned that decisions will be made and advice given that may be skewed by financial considerations. In the US, for instance, the overuse of MRI scans has been linked to the fact that many scanners are owned by doctors who refer their own patients to them for unnecessary scans.[26]

As for fraud on an industrial scale, there is no lack of evidence and many of the companies moving in on the NHS have already been successfully indicted in the US. A comprehensive account of cases brought and eye-watering fines paid is outside the scope of this book but the interested reader will find plenty of material. Of course monitoring fraud and pursuing it through the courts costs money which is lost to frontline care. In the US healthcare fraud is well recognised and dealt with by the FBI among other government agencies.[27]

Here in the UK we are babes in the wood and it is unclear how the NHS, in thrall to commercial confidentiality and struggling financially, will even know when it is the subject of serious fraud.

Cherry picking

Private companies have only one legal requirement and that is to make a profit for their shareholders. They are therefore anxious to avoid risk and unprofitable activity, which in health care means choosing straightforward low-risk patients whenever they can. High cost patients – typically emergency patients and those with multiple, complex and/or chronic problems – mean lower profits, and the private sector will when possible make sure the NHS has to deal with them.

The cherry picking of low-risk high profit patients by the private sector means that the NHS bears the cost of the difficult patients while the private sector makes its profits from the straightforward work, a pattern seen repeatedly when public services are outsourced – profits are privatised while risk is socialised.

Cherry picking first came to light when Blair's Labour government set up Independent Sector Treatment Centres (ISTCs) to deal with long waiting lists. Unlike NHS hospitals (paid per case treated for elective work) ISTCs were paid by block contract for a pre-agreed case load over five year periods, regardless of how few patients they treated. The more patients who could be turned away, however spurious the reason, the higher their profits would be. There was abundant anecdotal evidence that ISTCs were refusing to deal with unprofitable patients, for example with the elderly, the obese and patients with additional health problems, however trivial. There were stories of patients with previous mental illness or a history of drug misuse being turned down for routine surgery.

In a landmark paper (2009) Pollock and Kirkwood showed that ISTCs were indeed referring the difficult, i.e. unprofitable, patients back to the NHS and they calculated that the taxpayer had paid up to £3m for patients referred to ISTCs who had never received any treatment.[28]

When the Health and Social Care Bill was published concerns were expressed that with the greater role of the private sector would come a danger of increased cherry picking.[29] The government originally promised there would be safeguards against it in the legislation but the plans to pay a reduced rate for treating less complex patients were quietly shelved.[30] A Department of Health spokesperson said: 'We are committed to preventing cherry picking but there is more than one way to tackle this.'[31] They didn't go on to provide any details, nor have they become apparent since then. Indeed, as one writer pointed out,[32] since the HSC Act allows private companies to apply commercial confidentiality clauses to their NHS contracts it is highly unlikely that we will ever know whether and to what extent they are cherry picking patients.

NHS – the dumping ground

Since the private sector's aim is to maximise profits it is quick to avoid unprofitable patients or to return them to the NHS whenever possible. The cherry picking of NHS patients is one end of a spectrum of behaviour that runs right through to dumping sick patients in NHS A&E departments, as documented in the CHPI report. Dr Max Pemberton, in his article 'Superior private health care is a myth', recounts his personal experience working in an A&E department in central London where it was common to see acutely unwell patients arrive from nearby private hospitals and clinics, often 'without any proper hand over notes or details of the procedures that had been carried out'. Most of the hospitals didn't even have an ambulance to take the patients to an NHS hospital, but relied on dialling 999.[33]

Providing emergency care is expensive which is why the private sector would rather leave it to the NHS. As the CHPI report uncovered, many private hospitals have limited out of hours medical cover and little in the way of resuscitation teams or intensive care facilities. In 2007 an NHS patient died in an ISTC during routine gall bladder surgery after he had a haemorrhage on the operating table. There weren't enough swabs to stop the bleeding, and no emergency blood was stored, scandalous omissions by any standards. There was no phone in the operating theatre and eventually a porter was sent by taxi to the local NHS hospital to collect blood. When he arrived back with it two hours later it was too late.[34]

When the coroner criticised the clinic involved they replied 'We met all the criteria and all the regulations. (Blood) was not a requirement.' It turned out that the private sector, even when operating on NHS patients, was not offering the same checks and safeguards as the NHS because to do so would cost money. The NHS does what is necessary to safeguard patients; the private sector may do only what is stipulated in the contract, which in this case was not enough.

One of the most egregious cases involving the NHS being left to pick up the pieces was the breast implant scandal. In 2012 a French company, Poly Implant Prosthese (PIP) was discovered to have saved millions of euros by using industrial grade silicone (meant for mattresses) instead of medical grade silicone in their breast implants. Their prostheses were more prone to rupture and when the story appeared 47,000 British women were found to have received the implants, mostly for cosmetic reasons. Women who had had the operation on the NHS, mainly for reconstructive surgery after cancer, were offered free operations to remove and replace them.[35]

The government announced that it expected private clinics involved to offer the same deal, but they dragged their feet. Some had closed down, others refused to remove the implants for free until forced to do so. The Harley Medical Centre, facing legal claims from 1,700 women, went into administration to avoid being sued, transferring its doctors and clinics to a new company where it could continue its cosmetic surgery business without the threat of legal action. The multi-millionaire CEO, Mel Braham (who initially denied having a secret offshore company linked to the clinic) claimed that the Centre could not afford to offer free replacements to their patients, and demanded the NHS pay for the bulk of the costs.[36]

A spokesperson for the clinic said: 'The Harley Medical Group has always put patient care at the heart of everything we do. In response to [the implant scandal] we have acted in the best interests of our patients.'[37]

One of their patients was less impressed: 'I got a letter this week saying Harley was going into administration and that was the end of my claim. Harley was great when I was paying but now that the firm isn't getting money it's not interested.'[38]

Fearful women naturally looked to the NHS. The total NHS bill for dealing with affected patients, including those the private sector had turned its back on, was estimated at £3m.[39]

Terminating unprofitable contracts
Despite the incentives given to private companies it has proved difficult for many of them to make a profit from the

NHS, which is not surprising, given the very cost-effective nature of the public service they are seeking to replace. Since their business is to make a profit, companies may decide to terminate an unprofitable contract with the NHS, an option clearly not open to the NHS itself however 'unprofitable' delivering health care may be (just because something isn't profitable doesn't mean it isn't essential).

There is already a history of the private sector terminating NHS contracts, well-illustrated by the sorry story of primary care in north London. United Health Europe* first appeared on the NHS scene in 2003. In 2008 they bid for three GP practices in Camden and won the contract against a bid from local GPs on the 'value for money' score, despite the fact that the local doctors were judged to be offering 'superior core services'.[40] But in 2010, after recording an overall loss of £13.9m in the UK health market, United Health (UH) decided to pull out of primary care, anticipating that there would be more money to be made in providing commissioning support services to the newly forming CCGs. They sold the contract on, along with five other practices, to The Practice plc, 'the UK's largest operator of privatised NHS GP practices'.[41]

Camden Primary Care Trust (PCT), responsible for awarding the original contract to UH, thought it had contractual safeguards in place to stop the subcontracting of GP services but legal advice found otherwise. National rules allowed for contracts to be passed on without even the need to consult the PCT.

Worse was to come. In 2012 patients at one of the practices (142 Camden Road) discovered via their local paper that their GP practice was about to close. The Practice PLC explained that this was because its loss-making activities were

* Recently rebranded in the UK as Optum to escape the reputation of its parent company in the US.

169

'unsustainable'. At this stage it was being run by locums, had 4,700 patients depending on it, who were thus thrown on the mercies of adjacent NHS practices. Local GPs complained that the process had been chaotic, and that pat-ients' records had not been transferred. They also had worrying concerns that patients arriving from the Camden Road practice had received 'appalling care' and 'were often on the wrong medication'. Sorting out the mess was time consuming, time that had to be taken away from their own patients.[42]

The result of outsourcing this practice had been disastrous. Within four years a well-regarded and stable NHS GP practice (dating from the 1920s) had become a privatised business, to be traded on and then closed down when deemed unprofitable, changing hands twice in the process. 4,700 patients were left without a GP at very short notice. The much vaunted concept of 'patient choice' had played no part in the events and indeed patients had not only had no choice but had to turn to the local paper to find out what was going on. (The PCT bizarrely confessed that it had consulted only a few patients on the planned closure 'in order to avoid a run on other practices'.[43]) The patients were the last people who had benefited from this intervention by the private sector, while the companies involved had run rings around the NHS commissioners.

Camden Council's health scrutiny committee fought hard to hold an inquiry. They were highly critical of the contract and the lack of accountability and transparency, having had to use FoI requests in order to see the original contract. They reported: 'The contract was inadequate; it couldn't prevent UH from upping sticks and handing over to another provider. It makes a farce of the whole tender process.... In our view primary care by GPs should not be a commodity traded in the private market ...'

Neither UH nor The Practice plc deigned to attend the enquiry. *The Guardian* reported that the PCT had since amended its contracts, but given the private sector's access to high level legal expertise it is likely that they will continue to stay one step ahead of public services when it comes to writing favourable contracts.

Local GP Dr Paddy Glackin said: 'I don't think there is a single private operator that has seen out the full length of its contract to run a GP surgery in inner London. They cannot deliver the practice at NHS prices.' A UnitedHealth spokeswoman said that the Camden Road surgery was 'nothing to do with us anymore'.[44]

The Practice plc has form in this matter. The same *Guardian* article reported that they had terminated primary care contracts in Woking, Leicester and Nottingham. The accusation levelled against them was always the same – promises to invest while they were bidding for contracts followed by a failure to deliver (including the excessive use of locums[45]) and then walking away when there was no money to be made.

Other companies have behaved in the same way. In May 2014 Care UK pulled out of primary care in Newcastle half way through a contract after local campaigners complained about the quality of healthcare provision (see Chapter 4). The company left after 'reviewing (their) business strategy'.[46] In July 2014 Concordia Health asked to terminate their contract to run a GP practice in Kent.[47] By that stage the practice was staffed by locums, all of the permanent GPs having left within seven months of Concordia's takeover (a typical pattern after private takeover). There had been angry protests by patients concerned about difficulties in getting appointments, and lack of continuity of care after the departure of the permanent staff. The local NHS offered patients the unappealing alternatives of another company to come in and run the practice or registering with another.[48] Patient choice perhaps but not as patients had understood it.

In November 2014 Concordia pulled the plug on another contract in Dover two years early, leaving 3,650 'highly vulnerable' patients without a GP. The response of the NHS England spokesman is worth quoting: 'We feel that Concordia's withdrawal presents an opportunity to enable other GP practices to expand their patient lists, thereby becoming more resilient and better equipped to deal with challenges facing general practice ...' One local surgery showed their appreciation of this 'opportunity' by closing their patient list. At the time of writing the fate of the patients abandoned by Concordia is unknown.

In August 2014 Serco, one of the biggest players in NHS outsourcing, announced that it had experienced heavy financial losses on its NHS contracts and would be withdrawing from providing clinical services in the UK.[49] It said it would continue to bid for non-clinical services, presumably seeing its future and more money in helping to run the increasingly complex NHS market.

Perhaps it is worth asking in conclusion why the private sector is allowed to withdraw from unprofitable contracts while hospitals collapsing under the weight of unsustainable PFI debts cannot do the same?

The other unanswered question is whether the private sector can ever make a profit by taking over the running of a cost-effective health service without it resulting in deterioration in clinical services. The answer at the moment would appear to be not.

PFI — 'a total scandal, we've all been ripped off'

The predatory nature of the private sector in its dealings with public services is well illustrated by the ongoing saga of PFI. PFI has proved to be a costly disaster for the NHS with the financial problems of a number of trusts being traced to their crippling PFI debts (see Chapter 1), but one aspect of it that has received relatively little mention is the antisocial financial behaviour of the private companies involved.

In 2012 the *Sunday Times* drew attention to a report by the European Services Strategy Unit that 'as many as 270 PFI projects were based offshore avoiding millions in tax. These involve more than 70 NHS projects.'[50] Locating the firms off shore in places like Guernsey avoids payment of corporation tax and is logical behaviour by companies whose job is to maximise profits for investors — it is their duty to avoid tax whenever possible.

But it means that when taxpayers fund these NHS PFI projects the money is not recycled back into the UK economy but instead goes to tax havens abroad as well as into shareholders pockets. (Ironically one of the early arguments in favour of PFI was that taxpayers would benefit when the contractors paid UK corporation taxes). This looks even worse if you consider the large PFI profits already generated at the expense of the NHS budget, with the taxpayer set to hand over almost £80bn to PFI companies for £11bn worth of infrastructure. Margaret Hodge, chairwoman of the Commons public accounts committee, said 'it is shocking. Those who write PFI contracts should now insist the companies stay onshore.'[51]

But it seemed that once again few lessons were learned. In 2013 *The Independent* reported that private companies running NHS care services were using a tax loophole to reduce their taxable profits.[52] Margaret Hodge was again outraged:

> Companies have a duty to pay their fair share of tax ... Yet it seems every week brings a new revelation of another business that is using artificial structures to move profits out of the UK, seemingly for no purpose other than to avoid tax.
>
> The case of these private health companies ... I find particularly depressing. These are companies who get their income overwhelmingly from tax payers' money, for the purpose of providing a vital public service, yet do not appear to be making a fair contribution to the public purse.

The tax loophole in question had been put in place by the government, who had 'considered removing it' but then done nothing. In 2014 further evidence emerged about PFI financial sleight of hand at the expense of the taxpayer.[53] Private companies were doubling their PFI profits by selling on or 'flipping' projects a few years after finishing them, and just four big companies had made profits of more than £300m in this way. Many of the companies buying the contracts were based in tax havens which had been specifically set up by banks and fund managers for this purpose. PFI schools and hospitals were being 'flipped' as casually as pancakes and the companies concerned were pocketing the proceeds while the hospitals concerned, saddled with their massive PFI debts, were in increasing financial difficulties.

Margaret Hodge echoed the anger of her Tory predecessor Edward Leigh, who had described the refinancing of the Norfolk and Norwich Hospital PFI as 'the unacceptable face of capitalism'. She declared: 'It is a total scandal that the public sector has privatised these projects so badly. We have all been ripped off.' She conceded that many of the worst PFI cases had been negotiated under Labour: 'I'm afraid we got it wrong. We got seduced by PFI.'[54]

She complained that the government was bad at negotiating with the private sector, but after hearing so much evidence against PFI she failed to reach the obvious conclusion – that the problem was not that the government had privatised these projects 'so badly', but that they had privatised them at all. Complaining that the private sector maximises profits at the expense of public services is tantamount to complaining that cats kill birds. It is in their nature and the answer is not to try to legislate against the behaviour of cats but to recognise it and take appropriate precautions. No one would leave their cat in charge of the canary. Equally private companies cannot be trusted to behave well when delivering public services.

Anti-social behaviour – public v. private sector ethos

Public services are those which have been generally agreed to be so vital that their provision must be guaranteed.* It is clearly in our common interest to have universal provision in areas such as emergency services, law enforcement and education. In this country we have had the benefits of public provision of health care since 1948, and we have grown accustomed to a fair, universal and civilised system where we contribute according to our ability to pay and take out according to our need. Few people have any idea of the

---

* The European Commission, which calls them 'services of general interest', officially defines them in the following way: Services of general economic interest (SGEI) are economic activities that public authorities identify as being of particular importance to citizens and that would not be supplied (or would be supplied under different conditions) if there were no public intervention.

suffering that many endured from untreated illness before the advent of the NHS, nor is there a collective memory of the fear that people once had of the financial consequences of illness.

Public services are not profit seeking. Given their nature most public services cannot and will not generate a profit and as a result they are generally highly regarded because of their ethos. 'Patients before profits' has been the marching cry of NHS campaigners since the privatisation of the NHS began, and it neatly sums up the difference between the public and the private sector. As described above, the first duty of the private sector is to its shareholders and it shows. In December 2014 Margaret Hodge wrote about the outsourcing of public services:

> Too often contractors have not shown an appropriate duty of care in the use of public funds. Too often the ethical standards of contractors have been found wanting. It seems that some suppliers have lost sight of the fact that they are delivering public services, and that brings with it an expectation to do so in accordance with public service standards. The legitimate pursuit of profit does not justify the illegitimate failure to conduct the business in an ethical manner. A culture of revenue and profit driven performance incentives has too often been misaligned with the needs of the public who fund and depend on these services.[55]

The malign effects of privatisation on those who provide health care are insidious and multi-faceted, as the corruption of the 'industry' in the USA demonstrates. The medical profession no longer offers an intellectual leadership or the example of social conscience informed by science and humanity. The professional covenant with the patient is reduced to explicit contracts. Doctors become mere sessional functionaries.[56] Loyal company men and women, whose prime responsibility is to their employers, deny patients treatments that do not make a profit while, as front office salespersons, they recommend interventions that may not be in the patient's best interest (if their patient can pay). Medicine as a 'business' places the responsibility on its practitioners to shift as much product as can be paid for. (In the US even those who can pay have problems with excessive and/or unnecessary treatment, while those who can't go without.)

This chapter and the next are full of examples of failures of 'ethical standards' and of the profoundly antisocial behaviour of some private companies in pursuit of profit at the public's expense. We hear very little of this from the proponents of outsourcing public services, and when it is uncovered their conclusion is not that we need less of it but, as Margaret Hodge has recommended on more than one occasion, that we need to regulate it more tightly – something that has proved impossible thus far. The kind of regulation that would make the private sector more accountable and truly committed to meeting the needs of the population is at odds with the ethos of the multinational healthcare providers who are currently taking over more of the NHS.

New examples of unethical behaviour appear on a regular basis, and one was revealed recently when BUPA was found to have been offering patients bribes of £500 to £2000 to have their operations on the NHS rather than in their private hospitals. A letter to a cardiac patient explained 'If you are admitted to hospital under the NHS as an in-patient for any of the above procedures (cancer, heart and gynaecological operations) we will pay you a fixed sum amount'. Dr Clive

Peedell, a cancer specialist, accused BUPA of cashing in on the NHS. 'It looks as though BUPA have calculated that it's cheaper for them to pay patients to use the NHS than fork out themselves for private treatment which would cost them thousands of pounds.' A BUPA spokeswoman denied that the cash offers were bribes and claimed it was simply about 'offering customers choice'.[57]

The private sector is not above scaremongering to increase business. In 2013 bestmedicalcover.co.uk, a private medical insurance company, launched an advert which wrongly claimed that the English NHS had been responsible for 13,000 needless deaths since 2005. They misquoted Sir Bruce Keogh on the subject and went on to advise readers to prevent their health being part of the scandal, adding that 'health insurance could quite literally save your life'.

The Advertising Standards Authority received 54 complaints, which it upheld, judging that the claims made by the company were misleading and 'appeal to fear to sell private health insurance and that it was not justified to do so'.[58] Even so the advert had undoubtedly done damage by frightening people before it was withdrawn, with no possibility to correct it.

Private companies are also not averse to drumming up demand for unnecessary investigations when it stands to profit from them. In 2013 the *BMJ* reported that Specsavers, who had won thirty contracts to provide community audiology services, were sending leaflets to patients urging them to ask their GP to refer them to Specsavers for 'free' tests and hearing aids ('free' of course meaning paid for by the NHS). The invitation was also placed in newspapers and on buses. CCGs raised the alarm, saying that the drive was likely to stimulate unnecessary demand, eating into an already tight NHS budget. Dr Nigel Watson from the BMA's GP committee, called it 'the ugly side of commercialism', but Specsavers claimed it was their job to give patients 'access and choice'. And not to worry about who had to pay for it presumably.[59]*

Serco

One name crops up repeatedly in any discussion of the outsourcing of public services. Serco, once referred to as 'the biggest company you've never heard of', is now quite well known to the public and for all the wrong reasons. Since successive governments began outsourcing public services its name has appeared with monotonous regularity in UK headlines, associated with such poor practices as overcharging, falsified figures and a culture of 'lying and cheating'.[60] A closer study of Serco provides a useful example of private versus public ethos and what can go wrong when public services are outsourced to large supranational corporations.

Ninety per cent of Serco's global business is with public sector organisations, with 60 per cent of that business coming from the UK, where it is involved in an astonishingly wide range of activities including prisons, public transport, school inspections, 'Boris bikes' and the UK's ballistic missile early warning system.[61] It is what John Harris, in an excellent article, refers to as a 'public service company',[62] operating a parallel state.

Serco entered the UK health market in 2006 with a five-

*As for screening, in the private sector the sky is the limit. The author's then twenty-year-old son received an invitation from Life Line Screening to have an ultrasound scan to exclude arterial disease including abdominal aortic aneurysm. The letter promised 'You're in safe hands with Life Line Screening' – unless that is you are invited to pay £149 to screen for conditions you are extremely unlikely to be suffering from until late middle age.

year contract to run GP out of hours (OOH) services in Cornwall, having won with a bid that undercut the local GP co-operative by £1.5m. The contract was renewed in 2011, but in 2012 the service was severely criticised by the Care Quality Commission after whistleblowers drew attention to problems with understaffing and data falsification. In 2013 the Public Accounts Committee published a critical report accusing Serco of 'bullying employees, providing a short staffed and substandard service and manipulating data to hide the truth'.[63] The company admitted to having buffed up its performance data by altering them on 252 occasions in order to meet targets.[64]

The report was also critical of the local NHS authorities who had failed to negotiate a good contract, failed to scrutinise Serco's performance and failed to penalise Serco or terminate the contract when problems were revealed by whistleblowers. The report commented that Serco had consistently failed to meet national quality standards, and that the service was still not satisfactory despite the earlier CQC report. Margaret Hodge noted: 'The failures ... matter because the NHS will be making increasing use of private and voluntary providers to deliver NHS services.'[65] In the face of this evidence one might reasonably ask why, but apparently nobody did.

Serco said they were 'deeply saddened and very sorry' for what went on in Cornwall and in December 2013 announced that they had agreed to early termination of the contract after experiencing 'some operational challenges'. Valerie Michie, managing director of Serco's healthcare business, summed up with the immortal words: 'The services we deliver in Cornwall ... are no longer core to the future delivery of our healthcare strategy.'[66]

Despite this record, in March 2012 Serco won a £140m contract to deliver community health services in Suffolk after undercutting the incumbent trust by £10m. There were immediate fears that Serco had underestimated the true cost of running community health services, and these were soon borne out when Serco rapidly announced plans to cut 137 jobs out of 700 (proposals which were challenged by unions who threatened legal action). The local CCG subsequently identified numerous problems including inappropriate workload, lack of equipment, poor infection control, high stress levels and low morale among staff as well as recruitment difficulties.[67] In 2013 the *HSJ* reported that Serco was even appealing to the local NHS to help it fill vacant posts for nurses and physiotherapists, a request that was turned down.[68] NHS staff that moved over to Serco were relatively protected but new staff were given inferior contracts and struggled to manage the workload as staffing levels fell.

The GP commissioners proved tougher than their colleagues in Cornwall and began imposing financial penalties after Serco failed to make adequate improvements, although the money was to be restored once an action plan was agreed. A report by the CCG found that 'most frontline staff still state that they have no understanding of where the organisation is going and what needs to happen or change to get there'.[69] Serco continues to run this contract until 2015, but has said they will not bid to renew it. Meanwhile they pulled out of a contract to run Braintree Community Hospital in Essex.

Elsewhere Serco was branching out into the pathology business with two NHS London trusts – yet another tale of substandard service, low staff morale and overcharging described in Chapter 9.

Eventually the government had to act and in 2013 Serco

was barred from bidding for new contracts until it cleaned up its business. But in May 2014 they were back again and winning contracts *despite* still being under investigation by the Serious Fraud Office. A poll run by Survation at this time reported that the public had had enough. 80 per cent of the public thought Serco should not be allowed to bid for public service contracts, and had low levels of trust in outsourcing companies in general.[70] In August 2014 Serco had also had enough and announced it was pulling out of the clinical health services market in the UK, having lost £18m.[71]

The woeful tale of Serco's misadventure into NHS clinical services embodies many of the concerns around outsourcing. Overambitious bids were followed by an inability to deliver, data falsification, overcharging, poor treatment of staff,[72] a substandard service for patients and finally departure when profits were not forthcoming. The contracts were poorly drawn up – Margaret Hodge noted that in Cornwall 'you had the absurd situation where a company was seemingly lying about what it was doing but there was nothing in the contract that could allow you to terminate it – indeed they still appeared to be eligible for their bonus payments'.[73]

She went on to identify the problem at the very heart of outsourcing NHS services when she noted that such companies were 'good at winning contracts but too often they're bad at running services'.[74] Indeed, where tendering is concerned the level playing field promised by the government is a myth because the core business of these multinational companies is winning public sector contracts. They have the knowhow and legal expertise plus deep pockets for loss leaders, all of which gives them the advantage over charities, social enterprises and NHS staff who the coalition suggested would be in with a chance when it came to competing for

NHS contracts. Having won the contract they must then deliver a service of which they may well have no previous experience, with predictably poor outcomes.

Destabilising the NHS

In this chapter we have already had examples of contracts awarded to the private sector leading to destabilisation of local NHS services and there are a number of reasons why this may happen. It might be because the NHS is left to discover and then deal with poor outcomes for NHS patients who have been treated by a private company, as with the patients who had problems after joint surgery in the private ISTC. It may be because a private firm has abandoned a contract and left patients without cover, as happened after companies walked away from unprofitable contracts to run GP surgeries. It may be because the outsourcing of profitable services may leave an NHS unit unable to deliver the rump unprofitable service, as is threatened when MSK services are cherry picked leaving the local trusts with only the acute and emergency orthopaedic work.

The latest and perhaps most worrying example is unfolding in Nottingham where last year the local CCG awarded community dermatology services to Circle. The dermatologists at the local hospital, which had bid unsuccessfully for the contract, were reportedly concerned about job stability under a private employer, and also feared that Circle would not offer opportunities for training and academic research. The CCG ignored their concerns and six out of eight consultant dermatologists have since left, five citing their unwillingness to work for Circle. This means Nottingham University Hospitals Trust, until recently a national centre of excellence for dermatology, is now unable to offer acute and emergency adult dermatology services, an extraordinary and potentially dangerous situation by any standards.[75]

The British Association of Dermatologists (BAD) warned that the privatisation and fragmentation of specialist services was 'decimating' some areas of the NHS. Dr David Eedy, president of BAD, said an increasing number of private providers were taking on dermatology services around the UK, including in Cumbria and Colchester. He added that the exodus of staff should have been predicted:

> Nobody has thought through the implications for teaching, training and research – the whole future of British dermatology. Nottingham is just one example of the many fires we are fighting across the UK to try to keep dermatology services open in the face of poorly thought out commissioning decisions, and the Government's lack of understanding of the implications of pushing NHS services into unsustainable models provided by commercially driven private providers or enterprises.[76]

NHS hospitals are complex organisations whose many departments are interdependent to a high degree, which is often not appreciated by non-clinicians. They resemble children's Jenga towers in as much as removal of one block may lead to instability while the removal of too many blocks will inevitably lead to the collapse of the structure. Not only are different specialities dependent on the clinical expertise of many others (for example obstetricians and paediatricians must work closely together) but within departments expensive work has traditionally been cross-subsidised by simple and easier work. Thus NHS services will be destabilised if specific expertise is removed or easy work is outsourced. In Nottingham this has happened with fatal results for acute adult dermatology. Consultant dermatologists are in short supply, with 200 posts unfilled across the country, and it will be no easy matter to rebuild this department. NHS specialist teams, representing years of expertise, are like Humpty Dumpty – easy to break up, nigh on impossible to put back together again.

Conclusion

By 2013 outsourcing scandals were becoming commonplace, with ten separate investigations taking place (seven of them involving Serco) into services ranging from OOH GP services to housing for asylum seekers. It emerged that neither the Cabinet Office nor any other department knew how much public money was being spent on outsourcing and Margaret Hodge asked the National Audit Office (NAO) to look at government outsourcing, They chose to concentrate on four major companies (Atos, Serco, G4S and Capita) because of the scale of their work, their notoriety, and the criticism they had attracted.

The NAO report highlighted the fact that the government was outsourcing most contracts to a small number of firms, and Margaret Hodge voiced 'big concerns' over 'quasi monopolies that have sprung up in some parts of the public sector'. The report also drew attention to a number of other problems which will by now be familiar to the reader – lack of transparency over profits and outcomes, failure to pay corporation tax, overbilling, a culture which did not tolerate whistleblowers and the inability of small contractors to compete with the multinationals.[77]

Unfortunately their conclusion was not that the widespread

outsourcing of public services was an expensive way of getting a substandard service but that there should be better monitoring and stricter financial penalties. In other words, more public money should be spent on making the private sector clean up its act and behave more ethically, something which has been nigh on impossible to achieve so far. The elephant-in-the-room question that remains unanswered by all these committees and reports is – why is the solution to failed outsourcing more failed outsourcing?

The record of the private sector delivering NHS care is not a happy one. Because of the triumph of 'commercial confidentiality' hard data is hard to come by, but there is already plenty of evidence of worse outcomes for patients, unethical behaviour and poor value for the taxpayer, a complete contradiction of the claims made by supporters of private sector involvement. Meanwhile the NHS, criticised in the past as a monopoly provider, is in danger of being replaced by a small number of quasi monopoly providers.

It is easy to see how companies this big, winning the majority of public sector contracts and delivering vital public services, could become indispensable. *The Daily Telegraph* once suggested that 'without Serco, Britain would struggle to go to war'. Given what we know (rather than what politicians tell us) it must be equally dangerous to allow the NHS to rely heavily on expensive, substandard, unaccountable, cost-cutting and sometimes unethical and fraudulent private delivery to the extent that the purveyors of it, like the banks in the financial crisis of 2008, become 'too big to fail'.

The vexed question of 'public sector ethos' remains largely unaddressed. If the market is an inadequate guarantor of provision, then it is also inadequate as a motivator for people working in outsourced services. Outsourcing provision to profit-making firms, while keeping funding in public hands in order to resolve problems of market failure, raises the interesting problem of how people working in outsourced sectors are supposed to be motivated. Are they expected to work to public-sector ethos, while the firms for whom they work are profit-driven – with resulting tensions? Or do they too become profit-maximisers and give up the public service ethos? Do they need to be encouraged to have a distinctive ethos that guides their striving for excellence, replacing the profit motive? How is pursuit of that ethos to be guaranteed, and what is to stop practitioners slipping back into idleness? It is a particular dilemma for healthcare professionals, whose duty of care is to the patient, but who may find themselves working for the private sector whose first duty is to shareholders and who act accordingly. It is regrettable that professional bodies such as the General Medical Council have largely failed to address this question, leaving doctors exposed to potential problems arising from the conflict between professional duty and commercial pressures from employers.

It is incumbent on the cheerleaders for outsourcing the NHS to prove their case that the private sector delivers better cheaper health care and they have simply failed to do so. In fact all the evidence is to the contrary – not only are the private sector more expensive and less efficient but they may come with unacceptable baggage – lack of accountability and antisocial behaviour including fraud and corruption. They take no responsibility for training medical staff and increasingly their activities destabilise local NHS services. So why does privatisation via outsourcing continue?

In their 2007 paper Woolhandler and Himmelstein asked: 'What's driving privatisation?' Since 'the evidence is remarkably consistent; public funding of private care yields poor results' they reasonably concluded that 'only a dunce could believe that market-based reform will improve efficiency and effectiveness'. One could be forgiven for concluding that our elected leaders are all dunces.

9

Myth: We are not privatising the NHS.

The NHS is not for sale, there will be no privatisation.[1]

Andrew Lansley

There is no privatisation agenda ... my party doesn't want that.[2]

Jeremy Hunt

You told us you were worried about privatisation through the back door. So we have made that impossible.[3]

Nick Clegg

Privatisation of public services takes place when the government either outsources those services to the private sector or transfers ownership of those services to the private sector. The coalition government is doing both of these. The fact that thus far it remains free at the point of use is irrelevant. Contrary to politicians' denials they are privatising the NHS.

The insidious process of privatisation began some years ago but has accelerated under the present coalition government. This is because their 2012 Health and Social Care Act was explicitly designed to hasten the process. The government is pushing ahead with the privatisation of the NHS via a number of different mechanisms. These include:

- The outsourcing of services to the private sector through 'commissioning' or buying care from companies (Any Qualified Providers) such as Circle, Serco or Virgin Care.

- Sale of services to the private sector (e.g. pathology, plasma services).
- The use of Private Finance Initiatives (PFIs) that use private money to build new buildings and infrastructure for which the state has to pay at inflated prices for thirty years or more.
- The creation of foundation trusts that are run much more like private businesses and have the ability to raise funding from expanding private beds and services.
- Allowing services to become 'not for profit' organisations such as social enterprises, cooperatives or mutuals and no longer part of the NHS and thus vulnerable to corporate takeover.
- Limiting access to certain services previously provided by the NHS.
- The creation of market mechanisms for the distribution of funding within the NHS (e.g. commissioning, payment by results mechanisms, the purchaser-provider split and so called patient choice policies).
- The reduction of the role of government in regulating health provision.

* * *

The NHS has become part of our national life. No p(
party would survive that tried to destroy it.[4]

Aneurin B

Our best loved institution

Politicians know very well that the NHS is the UK's best lo
institution, more popular even than the royal family.[5] Ni
Lawson may have scornfully described it as 'the closest thi
the English have to a religion' but another Tory MP was mo
accurate when he told *Newsnight*: 'We are all socialists in
funny way when it comes to the NHS.'[6] Whether they approv
or disapprove of the public's love affair with the NHS al
politicians recognise the truth of Bevan's observation that no
political party can afford to be associated with its destruction.

No accusation is more toxic or potentially damaging
than that of an intention to privatise the NHS, which is
why the changes that have been introduced by successive
governments over the last twenty or so years have been
dressed up with language meant to disguise their true agenda.
Politicians are most anxious to deny any move towards
privatisation and David Cameron, Jeremy Hunt, Andrew
Lansley and Nick Clegg have all denied that the Health and
Social Care Act would result in privatising the service.[7]

In July 2014 even the Department of Health felt it necessary
to respond to an accusation from Unite that the government
was privatising English health care.[8] They recycled the usual
justifications for the reforms – that they were 'necessary for
patients' and that they placed 'the financial power to change
health services in the hands of those NHS professionals
whom the public trust most, and (put) clinicians, rather than
politicians, in control of healthcare'. The claims rang hollow,
particularly as by this time the reforms had little support

beyond Westminster and tens of thousands of patients, along with the same trusted professionals and clinicians, had taken to the streets to protest against what the government was doing to the NHS.[9]

But these denials are pointless when the Tories have a record that speaks for itself. As early as 1982 Tory grandees John Redwood and Oliver Letwin wrote a pamphlet (which Redwood subsequently disowned),[10] in which they advocated privatising the NHS. Letwin* has long had a central role in developing Tory policy and was described as 'the Gandalf of the process' in the period leading up to the 2010 general election.[11] He rather gave the game away in 1988 when he wrote a book with the not too subtle title of *Privatising the World, a Study of International Privatisation in Theory and Practice*. He also (in)famously told a private meeting in 2004 that the NHS would not exist within five years of a Tory victory.[12] In 2008 Jeremy Hunt,[13] the current secretary of State for health, co-authored a book (*Direct Democracy: an Agenda for a New Model Party*) which contained the following statement: 'Our ambition should be to break down the barriers between private and public provision, in effect denationalising the provision of healthcare in Britain.'[14]

However, the privatisation of the NHS that the Conservative party so earnestly sought behind closed doors could never have been achieved by the traditional methods that were employed for other services such as railways and energy, that is by the mass sale of shares to investors and private companies who would then own and make a profit from the NHS. No political party has ever dared to flout public opinion

* Tory MP, previously head of the Privatisation Unit at Rothschild's in the 1980s, then in Margaret Thatcher's policy unit, currently Chairman of the Conservative Research Department and of the Conservative Party's Policy Review.

openly in that way, knowing that the majority of voters (84 per cent in one YouGov poll)[15] oppose privatisation of the NHS. Instead the process has spanned more than one government and has been insidious, achieving its ends by a number of means.[16]

What constitutes 'privatisation' of a public service?*

There is no doubt that the primary intention of the Health and Social Care Act was the accelerated privatisation of the NHS, an outcome elegantly predicted by Dr Clive Peedell in his article for the *BMJ*: 'Further privatisation is inevitable under the proposed NHS reforms.'[17] In the article Peedell debunks the government mantra that privatisation cannot be happening as long as 'care remains free at the point of delivery'. Although politicians consistently suggest otherwise, care free at the point of delivery and privatisation of the public service are by no means mutually exclusive.

Peedell quotes the WHO definition of privatisation of health care, which is straightforward and describes accurately what has happened since the passage of the HSC Act: 'a process in which non-governmental actors become increasingly involved in the financing and/or provision of healthcare.'[18]

His article then cites five further criteria for defining privatisation of public services:

- Divestiture or outright sale of public sector assets in which the state divests itself of public assets to private owners.
- Franchising or contracting out to private, for profit, or

* Unite has published an informative pamphlet on the privatisation of the NHS in England http://www.unitetheunion.org/uploaded/documents/ GuideToNHSPrivatisation11-10734.pdf.

not for profit providers.

- Self-management, wherein providers are given autonomy to generate and spend resources.
- Market liberalisation or deregulation to actively promote growth of the private health sector through various incentive mechanisms.
- Withdrawal from state provision, wherein the private sector grows rapidly as a result of the failure on the part of the government to meet the healthcare demands of the people .

Peedell goes on to explain how every one of these criteria would be fulfilled under the proposals in what was then the Health and Social Care Bill and demonstrates how the HSC Act was drawn up to contain all the levers needed to enable and hasten the privatisation of the NHS. Despite the coalition's earnest denials this is exactly what has happened.

The HSC Act was passed in March 2012 but the final piece of the privatisation jigsaw was put in place in early 2013 with the passage of the infamous section 75 (see Chapter 4). This piece of secondary or 'enabling' legislation in effect requires all NHS contracts to be put out to tender and thus flies in the face of firm promises made previously by coalition ministers, MPs and peers. In March 2012, for example, the emollient health minister Earl Howe promised that commissioners would 'be under no legal obligation to create new markets' and would 'be free to commission services in the way they consider best'. Andrew Lansley himself had written to all GPs to reassure them that Monitor 'would not have the power to force you to put services out to competition'.[19] With the passage into law of Section 75 it was clear that their promises were worthless and GPs began to wake up to the extent of the betrayal. Critics claimed this would produce a 'major extension of market principles in the NHS', in which view they were supported by legal advice that competition would become 'the norm for placing NHS contracts'.[20] GPs themselves understood the implications of the legislation only too well and the vast majority were soon predicting that the NHS would be privatised within the next five to ten years.[21]

Monitoring privatisation

Is this view overly pessimistic? It has been difficult to track the rate of privatisation of the NHS since the passage of the HSC Act as the government is naturally keen to hide the figures, and for all Cameron's promises of transparency and accountability there is no central record of the number of outsourced contracts. It has been up to campaigning organisations and others to monitor these, with Unite, the NHS Support Federation and the *BMJ* all producing figures. The campaign group The People's NHS has set up a site with an 'NHS privatisation counter' showing how much of the NHS the government has sold off since the HSC Act came into force.[22] In October 2014 they managed to project an image of the counter onto the roof of the Tory Conference, a brilliant coup which was widely celebrated on social media if not by their mainstream brethren.

In May 2014 the NHS Support Federation estimated that in the two years since the Act was passed there had been a 30 per cent rise in the number of NHS contracts put out to competitive tender with their value increasing more than three times to total £13.5bn.[23]

Even more worrying was that the majority of these contracts were being awarded to the private sector. Already in 2013, just one year after the enactment of the legislation, the *BMJ* reported that only two of sixteen contracts awarded since the government's section 75 regulations came into force had gone to NHS providers, with the remaining fourteen going to private companies.[24]

By 2014 the NHS Support Federation reported that 70 per cent of contracts awarded through competitive tendering were going to private firms.[25] In the light of this figure Unite denounced the 'explosion' of contracts going to the private sector and demanded 'an inquiry into the impact of the government's changes, looking at the cost to the NHS of the new contract culture in terms of the bidding process and associated costs, as well as service and staff cuts as companies put profits before patient care'.[26] The government did not oblige with any figures about the additional costs incurred by the new tendering rules, indeed almost certainly did not even have the information, the possession of which might prove very inconvenient. It is much easier to deny what's going on if you're not keeping track of it.

In December 2014 the *BMJ* obtained up-to-date figures via Freedom of Information requests, which showed that between April 2013 and August 2014 a third of all contracts had gone to the private sector.[27] The government claimed that this showed there was no cause for concern but campaigners disagreed. They pointed out that the private sector don't want most NHS contracts, as big contracts for acute care are not profitable. Private companies were actually winning a much higher percentage of contracts in the areas in which they were interested e.g. elective care (they are now responsible for 15-20 per cent of elective surgery, a cause for concern, including for those responsible for training junior doctors).[28]

The high number of contracts going to the private sector

is hardly surprising. Tendering for a large NHS contract requires legal expertise, time and deep pockets, advantages possessed by the health industry multinationals but hardly by small voluntary sector organisations and NHS staff. One GP practice reported spending £40,000 on tendering for a service they were already running only to see it go to a private company who could undercut their bid.[29] The exercise not only wasted a large amount of money but took 'a senior partner and manager away from the practice for a lot of time'. It is understandable that while a few entrepreneurial GPs are learning how to get involved in tendering, most aren't prepared to risk further loss of money and staff time which would be better spent on patients. This of course leaves the field open to the private sector.

Another doctor responsible for a sexual health clinic wrote a heart-rending blog describing how he and his staff had had to take three months away from clinical work to draw up a tender for their own services. He notes with regret that 'quality' accounts for only 40 per cent of the total value of the bid* and points out the crass stupidity of taking clinical staff away from patients to write a bid to tender against experienced businesses who could throw money and legal (but notably not clinical) expertise at the process. (As we have seen, the private sector is better at winning contracts than delivering them). The blog[30] is well worth reading in its entirely as a microcosm of the terrible waste of time and money involved in the compulsory tendering out of all services, and the gross unevenness of the so-called playing field. If patients, faced with lengthening waiting lists, knew that doctors' and nurses' time was being wasted in this way there would be a riot. At the time of writing, the staff of the

* Despite the fact that the government had promised there would be no competition on price.

threatened clinic still don't know if they have been successful in winning the contract, but they surely know that they lost several months of frontline clinical care while they were forced to write the bid.

Transferring ownership of NHS services to the private sector

Once the coalition had successfully pushed the necessary privatising legislation through they quickly got down to business. One of the first victims was the state-owned company Plasma Resources UK. Reliable and trustworthy plasma supplies are vital to a wide range of patients, including people with haemophilia, and the company had been set up in 2002 to safeguard UK plasma supplies after the emergence of Variant Creutzfeldt-Jakob disease ('mad cow disease') meant that UK plasma was considered unsafe. But in July 2013 the government decided to sell an 80 per cent share of the company to Bain Capital, a US private equity firm founded by failed Republican presidential hopeful Mitt Romney, and better known for being 'job destroyers' than purveyors of high quality blood products.[31]

Dr Eric Watts, an eminent UK haematologist and former vice-president of the Association of Clinical Pathologists, feared that the privatisation of the service would mean 'losing control of the supply of important treatments to market pressures'.[32] An early day motion tabled by Labour MPs Jeremy Corbyn and Frank Dobson claimed that without the state company: 'the UK will be left buying its own plasma on the open market where there are supply chain issues of the sort that saw horses being labelled as beef.'[33] And, they might have added, that gave rise to the problems with UK plasma in the first place. (The problems had resulted from 'reduced UK regulation of cattle feed processing' which had allowed the transmission of a brain disease of sheep to cows whence it proved transmissible to humans).

Dobson and Corbyn, along with medical experts, warned that 'penny pinching neglect of safety procedures in the collection of plasma may well lead to an increased risk of infection',[34] and Vince Cable himself, alerted by the concerns of experts, had to be reassured by a DoH spokeswoman that the 'sale (was) good news for patient safety, taxpayers and jobs'.[35] Dr Watts did not think the taxpayer had benefited, however, describing the sale as 'another gift from the UK taxpayer to the market' as '£540 million has been spent to establish a company being offered for sale at a suggested £200 million'.[36] The government preferred the advice of management consultants (Lazard and Ernst and Young) to that of medical consultants and the sale went ahead. As Will Hutton remarked in *The Guardian*, 'Who would consign the provision of blood plasma to such custodians? Only a fool, a knave or a Tory politician'.[37]

Along with the privatisation of UK plasma services successive governments have had NHS pathology services in their sights. The scene was set with the two reports on English pathology services by Lord Carter of Coles[38] (who deserves and will get a paragraph to himself later on). The reports called for major reconfiguration through consolidation of services, with Carter arguing that the £2.5bn spent by the NHS on pathology could be reduced if services were delivered by 'stand-alone pathology service providers', independent of the hospitals in which they were based. The warning signs were all there, with recommendations about 'creating greater choice ... with more contestability and greater plurality of provision'. Accepting these proposals not coincidentally opened the door to private sector involvement, which has advanced most rapidly in London with so called public-private pathology joint ventures.

Some of this began under the previous government, when Guy's and St Thomas' NHS Trust entered into a 50:50 joint venture with Serco, forming GSTS pathology, which took over the hospitals' pathology services in deals 'worth £800 million over the next decade'.[39] Then in 2010 King's College Hospital joined the enterprise producing a tripartite venture called Viapath.

Concerns about the new public-private arrangements emerged as early as 2012, when *The Guardian* reported that clinical and financial failures had been uncovered by the independent research group Corporate Watch. They described an organisation 'in turmoil', documenting 400 clinical incidents in 2011, including 'losing and mislabelling samples' at GSTS's St Thomas' labs. The service exceeded the agreed monthly turnaround times for tests 46 times in 2011, with critical risk levels breached 14 times. They reported that staff morale was at an all-time low and that the new managers 'appear more concerned with marketing than laboratory work'.[40]

The full report is well worth studying and makes alarming reading, describing among other things problems arising from malfunctioning IT systems, undertrained staff and consequent damage to patients (see also Chapter 8). What's more the NHS hospitals had made no profits from the venture but had to continue to give it financial support. Corporate Watch concluded:

Running a pathology service without involving pathologists does not sound like a blueprint for success. Contrary to the current government's frequent promises that its reforms will put medical practitioners at the centre of decision-making in the NHS, involving private companies like Serco seems to do exactly the opposite, giving more power to non-medical managers. GSTS has been going for less than three years and yet it has already, as promised, shown what involving the private sector will do to the NHS.

In 2014 Corporate Watch reported further concerns, this time that the company had been overcharging the NHS to the 'tune of £283,000 in a sample three month period'.[41] Once again there was evidence that staff cuts and lack of investment had left 'laboratories close to disaster'. Internal e-mails from senior doctors accurately summed up the core problem of outsourcing public services when they claimed the company had an 'inherent inability ... to understand that you cannot cut corners and put cost saving above quality'. The whole undertaking increasingly looks like the worse possible combination of a public-private venture, with the NHS taking the risk and the private sector apparently living up to its reputation of putting profits before patients.

Privatising primary care

For a long time traditional primary care presented a solid face against the private sector but a number of factors have combined to change that. The ability of GPs to opt out of out-of-hours care (which happened on Labour's watch) created a point of entry for private companies and some quickly took advantage. At the same time smaller companies like Concordia and larger ones like United Health and Virgin started to bid for and win GP practices, and in 2011 Dr Clare Gerada, then chair of the RCGP, predicted that private firms would be running 10 per cent* of practices by 2014.[42] Some of the problems that have already been encountered are outlined in Chapter 8.

But the HSC Act crucially brought other forces into play. It was clear from the outset that GP commissioning was going to be a big challenge for GPs. Many were already struggling with their clinical load and few had the knowledge, time or expertise to take on commissioning on this scale. Lansley's white paper anticipated that they would need support and mentioned possible input from local authorities, the third sector and ex-primary care trust staff, but this is not quite how it has turned out. The subsequent creation of Commissioning Support Units (CSUs) has given rise to the possibility that decisions about outsourcing could themselves be outsourced.

CSUs, regional bodies currently subsidised by the NHS, were created to support CCGs. There are nineteen of them, and together they employ nearly 9,000 staff with a turnover varying between £21m and £62m. They are supposed to be off the NHS books by 2016 and according to Bob Ricketts, director of Commissioning Support Strategy at NHS England, there is 'a lot of interest from commercial providers'. One person involved in negotiations was quoted as saying: 'It's a great opportunity for the private sector ... They're not big businesses but they are likely to be increasingly influential and control billions of pounds. William Laing, of Laing & Buisson, the healthcare analyst, said: 'I can imagine private equity groups are keen on running [CSUs]; and I can see that the NHS is probably keen on them being taken over. The government couldn't have made it clearer that the CSUs are going to become independent entities by 2016.'[43]

If the private sector takes over the running of CSUs,

* It has proved impossible to establish a figure. There is little or no government transparency about the rate of privatisation of NHS services.

making decisions on behalf of CCGs about purchasing care, then much of the NHS budget will be in the hands of private companies who will be free to purchase that care from other private companies. Given the secretive world of offshore arrangements and rapid changes of ownership and name it will be impossible to avoid a situation where the private sector is buying care from itself. The privatisation of the NHS will have come full circle, and Dracula will be in charge of the blood bank.

Meanwhile the government has put out a tender for GP administrative support services. At stake is a ten year £1bn contract, one of the largest NHS contracts ever offered. Big multinational companies like Serco, G4S, KPMG, Capita – and even arms manufacturer Lockheed Martin – have shown interest. The NHS is excluded from bidding. Christina McAnea of Unison said: 'For there to be no NHS body or in house option just reveals the truth about the agenda of this government, which is running hell for leather in privatising as much of the NHS as they can before the general election in May [2015].'[44]

At the same time community health services were being put out to tender and in 2012 Virgin Care (previously Assura Medical) won a £650m contract, the biggest of its kind at the time, to run community health services in parts of Surrey (see below). When the contract was delayed it is rumoured that the local MP, one Jeremy Hunt, stepped in to push it through.[45]

Private companies taking over GP practices, compulsory competitive tendering, the outsourcing of community care and GP administrative support services[46] and influential CSUs run by the private sector mean that the privatisation of primary care, once viewed as unimaginable, is well under way.

Privatising secondary care

While some of the concern about the tide of privatisation has been focused on primary care, there are significant inroads being made into the secondary care sector as well, where privatisation is advancing on several fronts. Hospitals, under severe financial pressures, are increasingly filling their beds with private patients and at least one hospital – Hinchingbrooke hospital in Cambridgeshire – has been franchised out lock stock and barrel to a private company, Circle. Other threats include the creation of 'mutuals' and the appearance of 'self-funding' patients.

The story of the private takeover of Hinchingbrooke hospital by Circle* has already been outlined in Chapter 1. Suffice it to say here that the extensive mythology surrounding the carefully-crafted PR image of Circle and its proclaimed 'success' is almost entirely bogus. The company was not and is not a genuine 'partnership'. It has appalling relations with many of the frontline staff at Hinchingbrooke, refusing to meet with unions or, in recent instances, refusing staff time to attend 'partnership' meetings. In the last NHS staff survey covering all trusts in England, Hinchingbrooke came in the bottom half on two thirds of the 28 key issues and in the lowest 20 per cent of trusts on almost half of them. Staff numbers have been slimmed down beyond the sustainable level, resulting in a high and rising bill for temporary staff to keep services running.[47]

Circle as a whole has never yet made a profit as a company, and its bijou, tiny private hospitals in Bath and Reading stay afloat only thanks to treating higher than planned numbers of NHS patients. Its ten-year contract at Hinchingbrooke

---

* This chapter was written before the events of January 2015 mentioned in Chapter 12.

has not yet generated any profit, but has run up increasing deficits.[48] At the last count the company was just £185,000 short of the £5m level of investment in the Trust's balance sheet that could force a renegotiation of the deal, or allow Circle to walk away for a further payment of £2m. At one stage Circle were caught selling off hospital land to 'make the site more efficient'.[49]

Of course there are other ways of privatising secondary care apart from handing a hospital, its assets and a guaranteed revenue stream to a private company. One of the central planks of the HSC Act was the raising of the cap on the non-NHS income that foundation trusts could generate, including from private patients. The private patient income cap (PPI) was originally a sop from Tony Blair to prevent a backbench rebellion over the foundation trust legislation. It was based on the proportion of income from private sources at the time of becoming a foundation trust and had traditionally been very low – typically 2 per cent, apart from a few specialist hospitals, mainly based in London and with an international reputation.[50]

From October 2012 this figure was dramatically raised to 49 per cent for foundation trusts. While a few commentators were happy that it would give 'enterprise' in the NHS 'a freer rein'[51] the majority saw it as a major step forward in the privatisation programme[52] and a threat to an equitable NHS. The raising of the cap came against a background of financial problems for NHS hospitals – static budgets, reduced tariff prices for treatments and efforts by CCGs to save money by diverting patients away from hospital care. By the beginning of 2014 most foundation trusts were in deficit, with 66 (80 per cent) ending the most recent quarter with a combined deficit of £212m, the first deficit in the foundation trust sector's history. In September 2014 *The Guardian* reported that another 33 NHS hospital trusts expect to end 2014-15 with a combined deficit of £563m.[53]

Meanwhile bed numbers have been cut, and in April 2014 an OECD study reported that only Sweden had fewer hospital beds per capita than the UK.[54] The result has been longer waiting lists[55] and thus an increased incentive for patients who can afford it to seek private treatment. At the same time the dire financial straits of most hospitals means trusts are under pressure to raise money by allocating more NHS beds to private patients. This has happened most noticeably in those trusts which were already established centres of expertise, such as the Royal Brompton and UCH, which both significantly increased their private patient income by 37 per cent and 39 per cent respectively in 2013/2014. Foundation trusts are meant to re-invest any such profits in NHS care, but Dr Evan Harris in an article for *The Guardian*[56] noted that Moorfields Eye hospital had used its private patient profits to set up a branch in Dubai, where NHS patients are presumably unlikely to be found in the waiting room.

Ironically, at the same time that financial pressures are forcing the NHS to increase the number of hospital beds occupied by private patients, the government has also cut hospital bed numbers to the point where hospitals are having to buy extra capacity for NHS patients from private hospitals at inflated prices. In January 2014 *The Guardian* reported that Dame Barbara Hakin, deputy CEO of NHS England, was in discussions with private companies with a view to them providing 'spare capacity' in the event of a winter crisis (a revival of Alan Milburn's extravagantly expensive 'concordat' with private hospitals to treat NHS patients at up to 40 per cent above the standard NHS cost).[57] Using the private sector to bail out a struggling NHS is not unheard of for elective work, but this was an alarming development. The NHS Confederation reported that urgent and emergency care was on such a knife edge that 'hospitals may not be able to handle a sudden spike in demand'.[58] A DoH spokeswoman unhelpfully said 'we've increased the NHS budget in real terms but the NHS must also become more efficient if it is to meet the rapid rise in demand while ensuring compassionate care for all'. Professor John Appleby summed it up more truthfully when he said that hospitals could no longer 'maintain the quality of services and balance the books'.[59]

Once again the private sector was being proposed as the solution to NHS woes resulting from government mismanagement. The private sector was of course very eager to help out because their own income from patients with private insurance has been falling.[60] They are only too happy to plug the gap with NHS contracts and fill some of their many otherwise empty beds.

Mutualisation and 'self-funding' patients

Recently two other moves towards privatisation have appeared on the secondary care scene – mutualisation and 'self-funded' patients. Mutualisation has been touted by politicians and think tanks as a solution to the problems of the English NHS. It proposes that NHS providers be taken out of state ownership and managed by their employees, citing 'increased employee engagement' as one of the benefits. John Lewis and Arup are trotted as the enduring success stories but the list usually stops there.

Professor Martin McKee, in a recent *BMJ* article,[61] cites the many companies that did not fare well after mutualisation, including Northern Rock, Bradford and Bingley and the

Automobile Association, 'whose reputation plummeted after its new private equity owners cut costs, increased its debt and eventually walked away with £2bn profit'. He goes on to express concern that 'the journey to mutualisation ... could simply be the first step towards being swallowed up by a major corporation', a not unreasonable suspicion given the government's record, and wants to know how we ensure that these fledgling organisations remain mutual, and do not fall into the hands of asset-stripping private companies, based abroad where they are protected from demands for accountability and taxes. He points out that while mutuals have played a role in health care in countries like Germany this is because there are legal safeguards in place to stop corporate takeover, while similar organisations in England would enjoy no such protection. Mutualisation looks like yet another privatising policy wrapped up in cosy language and it must be regarded with a high degree of suspicion until and unless the safeguards McKee describes are put in place.

At about the same time that mutualisation was being enthusiastically promoted by the likes of Tory MP Francis Maude[62] news emerged of a new concept: 'self-funding'. In July 2013 a *BMJ* article[63] noted that a new category of private patient – the euphemistically named 'self-funding patient' – was being introduced at an increasing number of hospitals. These patients pay for their treatment – in NHS facilities or in private facilities delivering NHS care – at a rate based on NHS costs, which are typically considerably lower than those charged by private hospitals. Procedures available on this basis include imaging, ophthalmology services, and some surgical procedures such as hernia repair and arthroscopy that are now subject to 'restrictions' by CCGs and/or for which there are long waiting lists. As waiting lists get longer and more strictures are placed on what the NHS can provide the options available to self-funded patients naturally increase to fill the gap.

Those operating the scheme claim it allows 'patients to access restricted treatments at a cheaper rate than the private sector' but behind the spurious justifications it is, as John Appleby of the King's Fund has pointed out, 'paying privately to get some healthcare provided by the NHS. It is a private scheme.'[64] More importantly it blurs the boundaries between the NHS and the private sector, creating yet again the conditions for a two tier NHS in which it is inevitable that those who can pay will either queue jump through buying access to the service or will get treatments that aren't available to those who can't pay, or both.

Private provider Care UK is quite unabashed about it. A leaflet sent to GPs and patients, offering self-funding at four of its eleven NHS funded treatment centres, says: 'If you require treatment but cannot access it through the NHS you may choose to opt for Self Pay. This way you'll benefit from prompt medical care at a time that's right for you – and with Care UK it may cost less than you imagine.' Nick Hopkinson, a London consultant chest physician voiced the concerns of many when he said that he feared this would lead to queue jumping and an inferior service for those who couldn't pay, and that once 'the private providers have integrated themselves into NHS provision they'll be in a position to offer people their premium service as well'.[65]

It's not hard to see how insurance companies will step up to offer cover for those who would like to be 'self-funding' when the need arises, thus exacerbating this fundamental break with the concept of equity, one of the founding principles of the NHS.

Private companies are increasingly taking advantage of the fact that the boundaries between private and public are becoming more blurred. In another *BMJ* article[66] Margaret McCartney describes the private company Better as.one[67] which guarantees 'medical peace of mind' for £300 a year. For this relatively modest sum you the subscriber are entitled to an urgent triage by a consultant as soon as 'you have a condition that concerns you'. Thereafter you can be referred back to the NHS for tests and treatment which the company will help you access 'as quickly as possible'. As McCartney points out the offer of a 'fast track to treatment on the NHS' not only undermines the purpose of primary care as a gatekeeper but also means that the NHS pays to 'sort out non-evidence-based interventions that began in the private sector'. And once again patients who can't afford to pay to bypass the system will find themselves in the queue behind those who can.

Outsourcing

The introduction of compulsory competitive tendering has led to more contracts going to the private sector for the reasons described earlier in the chapter. This is happening in primary care, secondary care and in community services, and as the contracts become larger and more complex they increasingly span the boundaries between all three.

Many only woke up to the shape of things to come when, in 2012, Virgin Care was awarded a £650m contract to run NHS community health services in Surrey. The contract included community nursing, health visiting, physiotherapy, diabetes treatment and renal care, prison health care and sexual health services.[68] Losers in the bidding process were Central Surrey Health, the government's flagship social enterprise mutual, and a local NHS foundation trust, both of whom presumably had a little more clinical experience than Virgin. Virgin Care had recently taken over Assura Medical and went on to bid successfully for a number of other contracts. NHS campaigners remain particularly incensed at Richard Branson's forays into the NHS and have managed to temporarily close a number of Virgin shops with street protests.[69]

Further large contracts have since appeared, including, in 2013, an £800m contract to run integrated adult and older peoples services in Cambridgeshire which again includes acute and community services, and is set to run well into the next parliament. It met with much resistance from local campaigners[70] and was eventually (eighteen months later) awarded to an NHS consortium, with an estimated minimum £1m* spent on the procurement process – taxpayers' money that would surely have been better spent on patients than lawyers and accountants.[71]

The final straw for many came with the announcement that four CCGs in Staffordshire were putting together a contract worth £1.2bn for cancer services and end of life care.[72] The cancer care contract, worth £687m, is set to run for ten years and has attracted the attention of a number of private companies, who are being advised by Macmillan Cancer Support charity.** It is ironic that the CCGs involved say that they want a 'more joined up system' for their patients, given that it is largely the coalition's reforms that have led to the fragmentation of traditional patient pathways – another classic example of running down the NHS and looking to the

* Although rumour has it that the tendering process itself had cost up to £10m.
** Donors were not slow to express their dismay that a rumoured £800,000 of their donations to Macmillan were being spent on helping private companies bid for NHS cancer services.

private sector for the answer. The plan to contract out these services has triggered an impressive scale of opposition, with thousands signing petitions and hundreds attending public meetings and protests – a level of public engagement seldom seen before in campaigns against privatisation.

Paul Evans, director of the NHS Support Federation, commented: 'The most sensitive areas of NHS care are being opened to the private sector. This shows there is no limit to the willingness of the government to replace NHS services with those from profit-driven companies.'

Dr Clive Peedell, co-leader of the National Health Action Party and a cancer specialist, was concerned:

[T]here are already national shortages of professionals involved in cancer management. Contracts with non-NHS providers will take many of these highly trained staff away from the established NHS services, where the full range of cancer services are delivered to a regional population.[73]

He also noted that the project is being driven by the Strategic Project Team (SPT) – a shadowy part of NHS England with a history as 'arch privatisers'. The SPT – consisting mostly of management consultants rather than permanent NHS employees – have been involved in most of the 'ground-breaking' NHS privatisations to date.[74]

As in Staffordshire, the Coastal West Sussex Commissioning Group also cited concerns about joined up care when it handed a contract for orthopaedic work worth £235m to BUPA in September 2014.[75] It later emerged that the majority of the group who awarded the contract were unable to vote because of 'conflicts of interest' i.e. they presumably stood to gain financially.[76] The CCGs Declaration of Interest Register makes interesting reading and was criticised for not being up to date at the time of awarding the contract.[77]

According to the *Chichester Observer* the contract meant that local hospitals would no longer be responsible for orthopaedic services, although a 'local NHS spokesperson' disingenuously claimed that patient choice would not be affected (unless of course they chose to go to their local hospital). It is of course tempting to ask what will happen if the private provider decides to terminate the contract (as has happened previously, see Chapter 8) at which point the orthopaedic departments in the local hospitals will presumably have been disbanded and there will be no services at all to choose from.*

Private sector cheerleaders

The process of privatisation has also been helped along by the outsourcing of NHS policy decisions to private companies – the so-called privatisation of policy – and by the infiltration of the NHS by private sector cheerleaders. These are typically people who come from a private sector background to work in or advise the NHS and/or those with financial interests in the private sector who are appointed to positions of influence in the NHS.

Typical of the latter is Lord Carter of Coles, the Labour peer who founded Westminster Health Care and built it into a major healthcare provider, which he sold in 1999. His own biography says 'He is a private investor and director of public and private companies in the fields of insurance, healthcare and information technology'.[78]

In 2008 Lord Carter, (who also conducted the pathology

* The local hospital has already written to local GPS expressing serious concerns about the viability of local A&E departments if orthopaedic services are outsourced.

reviews mentioned above), was appointed as chair of the Competition and Co-operation Panel (CCP), in which position he was meant to 'ensure fairness when private-sector firms bid for public contracts'. In March 2012 *The Daily Mail* revealed that he had a number of well-paid positions with the same private firms which were bidding for NHS contracts, including chairman of the UK branch of the American healthcare firm McKesson (for which he had received £799,000 in the previous year). There were immediate calls for him to step down, including from Professor Clare Gerada,* who said, 'he cannot have any credibility when he is also heading a company with such huge interests in the very contracts his organisation is meant to police'.[79]

Another classic example is that of Sir Stuart Rose, former head of Marks and Spencer, who in February 2014 was appointed 'to lead a review into how to improve management in the NHS in England'. The BBC headline: 'Ex M&S Boss to Advise NHS Managers',[80] typically enquired no further but others were more curious and 4bitnews was soon reporting that Sir Stuart had some worrying conflicts of interest[81] in his new role. He was, *The Independent* reported: 'paid to sit on the advisory board of Bridgepoint, an international private equity group, which is the major shareholder of private healthcare firm Care UK. Care UK is in the running to take over the George Eliot NHS Hospital Trust – one of 14 hospital trusts in Sir Stuart's review.'

A DoH spokesperson hastened to reassure everyone that Sir Stuart 'committed to recuse himself from any relevant

* The article is worth reading in full because of the covert connections it reveals between some NHS officials and the private sector, and some interesting facts about McKesson's criminal record in the US, where its chief executive was jailed for one of the biggest corporate frauds in American history.

health discussions at Bridgepoint European Advisory Board meetings' but it didn't look good for transparency in the NHS.

There are many egregious examples of such conflicts of interest and the curious reader is referred to the NHS Support Federation website 'NHS for Sale',[82] which includes details of the revolving door between the public and the private sector as well as the financial interests of peers and MPs who voted on the HSC Act. The latest politician to pass through the revolving door between government and the private sector is Stephen Dorrell MP, until recently Chair of the House of Commons Health Select Committee. He took a job as a 'health policy consultant' with KPMG, and announced that he would be standing down at the general election as his new position would be 'incompatible' with his role as MP. He did not apparently see any problem with staying on as an MP until then, and there were immediate calls for him to step down, not least because KPMG was looking to bid for a £1bn NHS contract. Labour MP Grahame Morris referred him to the Commissioner for Standards for a possible breach of the Commons Code of Conduct and Dr Clive Peedell said: 'This case demonstrates everything that is rotten about our political system.' KPMG declined to reveal his salary but noted that 'his knowledge and expertise will be a huge help'.[83]

Another appointment that raised eyebrows was that of Lynton Crosby, hired as an advisor to David Cameron in 2012. His PR firm had previously advised businesses looking for NHS contracts, and Andy Burnham thought it was no coincidence that after his appointment the government announced new rules on tendering out all NHS contracts. *The Mirror* quoted Burnham:

Shortly after Lynton Crosby started work for the Conservatives, the Government shifted its position in favour of private health companies by trying to sneak NHS regulations through the House, forcing services out to the market. At the time, experts expressed surprise at the sudden shift. Now we can guess why. Once again, it is more proof that you can't trust David Cameron with the NHS.[84]

One the most alarming and insidious encroachments of the private sector into the NHS has been via the 'privatisation of policy making', much of which has involved the big management consultant firms. McKinsey (the Jesuits of capitalism) have for example been called the 'firm that hijacked the NHS' and they have been credited with undue influence at every level from coming up with the £20bn 'efficiency' savings to drafting the HSC Bill. A 2012 article in the *BMJ* – 'Behind closed doors: how much power does McKinsey yield?' – revealed the full extent of their penetration.[85] Former and current senior staff could be found in many influential positions including 'think tanks' like the King's Fund and the Nuffield Trust, as well as NHS bodies such as Monitor, and there is a revolving door between McKinsey and government departments[86] with consultancy staff on government secondment while 'civil servants leave to join consultancies they may previously have hired'.[87]

(More details of the web of connections between government, management consultants and the lobbying industry can be found in the appendix on the health lobbying industry).

We didn't vote for it and we don't want it

The term 'creeping privatisation' is now appearing in the media, but as ever they are behind with the NHS news. Under the coalition the process has accelerated from creeping to galloping and is now, to mix metaphors, advancing across the front lawn and kicking down the door. Despite the evidence all around us the media are still often surprisingly shy about using the word – even *The Guardian* still sometimes puts it in inverted commas as though there remained some doubt about it.[88]

In their excellent book *The Plot against the NHS,* Colin Leys and Stewart Player write: 'For 20 years successive governments have pursued a policy [for the NHS] that the public hasn't voted for and doesn't want.' The public has never voted for privatisation of the NHS and certainly doesn't want it. Poll after poll shows that the public does not want further involvement of the private sector and would be prepared to pay more for the NHS. According to a 2013 YouGov poll, 84 per cent of the public would prefer to see the NHS run as a not-for-profit public service, whilst just 7 per cent favour privatisation.[89] The latest poll shows 80 per cent of the public are ready to pay higher taxes to protect the NHS from privatisation.[90] And yet by all accepted criteria the coalition is proceeding with the privatisation of the NHS while denying what it is doing. Hundreds of GP surgeries are now owned by private companies and billions of pounds worth of contracts have been awarded to the likes of Serco and Virgin.

Chapter 8 has already examined why the private sector should not be delivering NHS care, and Chapter 11 will expose some of the reasons why privatisation is nevertheless still on the political agenda. In the meantime we must continue to explain to the public and the media that we are not, as ministers suggest, indulging in 'ludicrous scaremongering' but responsible truth mongering. We must use the 'P' word on every possible occasion. Privatisation is proceeding apace and will do irreparable damage to the NHS and our patients.

Will Hutton recently wrote an article in *The Guardian*, contrasting the public and the private sector. He accused the latter, exemplified by G4S and Serco, of having 'built a culture in which exploiting, rather than serving, the customer comes first'. The NHS on the other hand: 'still manages to combine humanity and efficiency. Its systems are not extravagant, but there is a sense, as I recently discovered with a close family member in a long spell in hospital, that the patient remains at the centre of everyone's preoccupations.'[91]

This is the precious quality we stand to lose when we privatise public services, in particular a service as person-centred as the NHS. The final warning comes from Professor Arnold Relman, the former editor of the *New England Journal of Medicine*:

The continued privatization of health care and the continued prevalence and intrusion of market forces in the practice of medicine will not only bankrupt the health care system, but also will inevitably undermine the ethical foundations of medical practice and dissolve the moral precepts that have historically defined the medical profession.[92]

10

More myths: There are no cuts, only cost improvements. Closures and 'reconfiguration' of services are clinically led.

We'll cut the deficit, not the NHS.[1]

David Cameron, election poster 2010

We were told that whilst we would lose our A&E, we would also gain all these excellent community services. Now they're planning to cut millions from their budget that would have been spent on community services. It's unfair on residents.[2]
Sharon Massey, Bexley council's cabinet member for health, February 2009

Despite David Cameron's pre-election promise to 'cut the deficit, not the NHS', cuts in health services resumed within weeks of the 2010 election, driven by the freeze on NHS budgets. By October 2014, 66 A&E and maternity units had been closed or downgraded along with the loss of 8,649 beds. One fifth of these were mental health beds, but most were 'general and acute' beds dealing with emergencies and waiting list patients, many of them older people for whom there is only restricted provision of social care after 27 per cent cuts in local government spending.

Cost-saving schemes in various hospital reconfiguration plans include reducing 'non-elective' admissions (i.e. emergencies and urgent referrals), as well as cutting numbers of A&E attendances, outpatient appointments, and even elective (waiting list) operations. So each of these 'efficiency savings' is in fact a planned *reduction* in the availability of services.

Many reconfigurations revolve around closure or downgrading of an A&E, even though A&E services represent only a very small share of NHS spending. However, closing A&E is often a first step to downgrading and closing hospitals.

No closure plans are ever honestly presented as cuts: they are painted up as 'reconfigurations' to centralise services in other hospitals, and treat patients 'closer to home'. But hardly any of the promised community-based or primary care 'alternative settings' for care actually exist, even on paper. There are no staff, no premises, no plans, no money and no political will to establish these services – which may well prove more expensive and less efficient than the hospitals they are supposed to replace.

The evidence for cost savings from developing GP and community out of hospital initiatives is very limited. In 2012 authoritative research challenged the received wisdom that hospital admissions could be reduced by improving primary care interventions, especially those aimed at 'high risk' patients.

Promising to locate more and more services in smaller community settings 'closer to home' makes good sound-bites, but hard questions need to be asked about the costs and efficiencies involved, and availability of essential but sometimes scarce professional staff. It's clear that most local communities have not been persuaded: campaigns continue against almost every cutback and closure.

* * *

Cuts, closures and plans for reconfiguration did not begin in 2010 with the Tory-led coalition government, but they have proliferated in the last few years and will continue to pose a threat to services until such times as the spending freeze is broken and serious fresh investment can match resources to local needs.

Already the impact has been considerable. In October 2014 the staunchly Tory *Daily Telegraph* published an updated list of the 66 A&E and maternity units that had been closed or downgraded since 2010,[3] or were still under threat, four years after David Cameron and then shadow health minister Andrew Lansley had toured the country promising to halt such closures and 'cut the deficit not the NHS'.

We all know that things have turned out very differently from the promises that were made by the Tories in opposition. Along with the A&E and maternity units that have closed, the period from 2010-14 has seen the loss of 8,649 beds – two thirds of them the frontline 'general and acute' beds which care for emergencies, elective admissions and older people. One in five mental health beds (1,693) are also among those lost, while mental health spending has been falling year by year for the first time in over a decade.[4] None of this was included among the pledges and promises as the Tories chided Labour for planned local cuts and posed in front of threatened hospitals, promising to save them if elected.

Indeed Tory justification for the 'reforms' and policies they have introduced has been to improve performance. But again reality has been very different. The reduced capacity, at a time of rising demand, has brought sharp increases in the numbers waiting (up almost a quarter since the 2010 election), waiting times, and numbers waiting over eighteen weeks for treatment (up 12 per cent). The percentage of patients waiting less than nine weeks for cancer treatment, which peaked at 88 per cent, has fallen below the 85 per cent target and well below the levels achieved in 2010. In January 2015, newspapers and other media were full of reports on increased waiting times in A&E departments.

Coming as it did after a decade of investment and improvement, the prolonged freeze on NHS spending imposed since 2010 has resulted in a decline in performance, while the cash constraints have opened up a new drive for cuts and closures – which are now discussed under the much less explicit heading of 'reconfiguration'.

Like many euphemisms, this buzzword is inherently misleading, since 'reconfiguration' implies that the same level and range of resources are being reorganised. In fact, whatever else people may claim, the bottom-line objective of reconfiguration is to make substantial and sustained reductions in spending.

It's all about the money

Dishonesty is at the centre of the presentation of plans for reconfigurations. Any suggestion that the gallons of red ink on financial spreadsheets are the real reason behind such reconfiguration plans, rather than a response to patients' needs, is always immediately and indignantly refuted. How dare we suggest otherwise?

These plans, we are told, almost always by some managerial bureaucrat with a straight face and increasingly lengthening nose, are certainly not financially-driven. They are claimed instead to be 'clinically-led' proposals to improve patient care, proposals that (they hope) just happen to cut costs. It's not clear if anyone at all believes this.

If anyone *does* believe it, it is clearly not local communities whose hospitals face a downgrade, loss of services or closure:

they are swiftly able to see through the rhetoric to the reality.* They are all too aware that the issue of whole populations facing longer journeys for treatment (or to visit relatives and friends in hospital) has been largely ignored. Time and again they find that the management consultants or senior NHS managers who drew up the plans either live miles away, or have comfortable cars to convey them wherever they want to go – and perhaps even private health insurance.

Of course, the managers driving these projects can never let on that they know that we know that what they say is at best economical with the truth, and based largely on wishful thinking. They plough on, spelling out proposals using a language which consistently misleads those who look simply at the words and not the essence of what is proposed.

A closer look at many of the plans reveals the true picture. In north-west London, for example, where one of the biggest-ever packages of cuts and closures has been proposed, the underlying aim is clearly a reduction in services to generate cash savings. The projection was a £1bn potential cash gap over five years, to be met by £553m of commissioner savings and a requirement for NHS trusts (those not yet foundation trusts) to generate savings of £360m over three years.[5] The cost-saving schemes (mapped out in a separate document from the hospital reconfiguration) fall into six main categories, all of which can also be seen in many other reconfiguration plans:

* The NHS Confederation has recognised this problem and produced a whole pamphlet written by spin-doctors, advising CCGs and trusts how best to push through their reconfiguration plans against the tide of local public opinion. It makes amusing reading. NHS Confederation (2014) *Reconfigure it out. Good practice principles for communicating service change in the NHS*, September, NHS Confed: http://www.nhsconfed. org/resources/2014/09/reconfigure-it-out-good-practice-principles-for-communicating-service-change-in-the-nhs.

- Cutting back on the contracts for acute, community and mental health providers. This is officially described as *Contract Management*.
- Diverting patients away from hospitals and existing services and moving them into 'lower cost settings of care' (many of which do not yet exist) and 'care closer to home' (also largely non-existent). This is officially described as *Changing setting of care*.
- Reducing overall numbers of patients accessing treatment – not necessarily the same as the much more complex issue of reducing the levels of medical need. In the jargon of NHS speak, this is *Reducing demand*.
- Changing the ways in which patients access services (again requiring investment and new services which have not yet been established). This is described by NHS bureaucrats as *Pathway redesign*.
- Corporate 'efficiency savings' through outsourcing, centralisation, shared services and the asset-stripping of estates. This is generically described as *Back office and corporate savings*.
- Savings from prescribing and medicine management, either by better use of generics, or by restricting access to more costly drugs and imposing limitations on GP freedom to prescribe. This is described officially as *Reducing drug spend*.

Behind the bland phrases, to which few could object on principle, come plans for very large scale cutbacks in hospital care in the next few years, which many object to in practice. In north-west London, for example, the plans aim to reduce hospital activity by:

- 19 per cent fewer 'non-elective' (i.e. emergencies and urgent referral) admissions to hospital. This is equivalent to 55,000 hospital admissions a year, and would open the way to close 391 hospital beds.
- 22 per cent fewer outpatient appointments – a massive 600,000 reduction in hospital appointments.
- 14 per cent fewer A&E attendances – 100,000 fewer to be treated.
- 14 per cent fewer elective (waiting list) operations – a reduction of 10,000.[6]

In other words each of these 'efficiency savings' is part of a planned *reduction* in the availability of services. This also raises questions about whether existing services that close would be replaced at all. Tucked away at the back of the document were projections of how many jobs (up to 5,000, most of them clinical posts) might be cut to generate the savings required.[7]

Of course all these savings also have a cost: the financial impact on local hospitals of cuts on this scale could throw the finances of already troubled trusts into crisis. According to figures produced for the 2007 Darzi report on London's NHS, in the north-west London example the non-elective cuts alone could cut hospital revenues by at least £330m, spending on outpatients by £60m, and elective services by another £40m – an overall cut equivalent to *20 per cent of the income of local trusts.**

Developments since then have demonstrated that the critics were right, and those driving the reconfiguration had no serious plans to replace the lost services and beds when A&E units and whole hospitals close: in north-west Thames,

* Calculations conservatively based on figures in Darzi, *Technical Report*, 2007.

just two months after the closure of the relatively small A&E units at Hammersmith and Central Middlesex, performance of the neighbouring hospitals in handling emergencies has plunged to the lowest levels anywhere in England. Trust managers at nearby Northwick Park Hospital, in the same trust as Central Middlesex hospital, have complained that bed numbers were inadequate as queues grow for treatment.[8]

Scratch the surface of almost any local reconfiguration plan, and a similar set of less obvious objectives and dubious assertions will emerge.

The deception begins on the covers of the documents outlining the plans: they invariably carry absurdly positive, happy-clappy titles that belie their real purpose. Many such titles have already been tried – *Shaping a Healthier Future, A Picture of Health, Better Care Closer to Home, Healthier Together, Investing in Excellence* … there are many more.

Somewhere in the bowels of NHS England or some management consultants' headquarters a title generator must be cranking out endless permutations of a few positive words to create a steady flow of vacuous reassurance. However, nobody is that easily fooled. It's instantly clear that none of these documents really means what the title suggests, and so the tactic is immediately counter-productive, since the unreality of the title annoys the plan's opponents rather than soothing them or allaying any fears.

Constructive use of boredom
The structure of such documents is always similar, and many of them appear to have been bolted together from ready-made pre-drafted sections from some restricted access NHS England website with only a few 'local' details thrown in.

That's why almost every consultation document begins

with at least 10-15 pages of general twaddle on public health. All that's needed is a series of truisms on national and local prevalence of disease, mortality statistics, smoking, drugs, alcohol and other health issues, deprivation, demographics, ethnic mix and inequalities. And of course a disquisition on the benefits of preventive health campaigns and the need to combat inequalities in health.

Anything will do, as long as it's dull and non-contentious. Nobody will be against any of it, but none of it bears any relation to the plans that are being proposed. The idea is to bore potential critics who may pick up the document, and persuade them there is nothing to get their teeth into.

However significant they may be in their own right, the data, the statistics, and the hopes to effect a reduction in hospital caseload through improving the health of the local population are not the real reason for change, or the basis for the plan. But including this information does have a purpose: it ensures that all the practical content of the document and any controversial plans or figures can be pushed to the middle, or to the back, of a document that will be frustrating to read for any but the most determined critic.

Despite the pages allotted to them, many plans in practice ignore the public health and health inequalities issues altogether when they get down to the real business of closing hospitals and services in the most deprived areas. This has been the pattern of proposed closures in north-west and south-east London.

The war on A&E

One feature which almost all reconfiguration documents have in common is a focus on downgrading or closing A&E services, often leaving only an Urgent Care Centre (UCC), so diverting all those with the most serious and urgent health needs much longer distances to centres elsewhere.

The rhetoric to conceal this involves two deceptions: misleading use of statistics showing lives saved as a result of centralising highly specialist services for stroke and trauma services (comprising less than 5 per cent of all A&E attendances)[9] on the one hand, while on the other arguing that an inflated proportion of current A&E patients who have only minor problems might be treated in primary care or in community services if they were ever to be made available. So far we have seen varyingly exaggerated claims ranging upwards from 60 per cent – with some saying 70 per cent, 75 per cent, 77 per cent or even 80 per cent of A&E caseload is so minor it could be dealt with on the same site in a scaled-down, nurse-led UCC, in conjunction with other services in 'community settings'.

The Special Administrator's plan for cuts in Lewisham

One classic example of this invention of ambitious statistics, in defiance of the evidence, can be found in the Trust Special Administrator's (TSA) plans for the closure of two thirds of the Lewisham Hospital site, its A&E and other services. Most of this hangs on the extravagant claim that only 23 per cent of the 115,000 patients a year attending Lewisham A&E would need to be treated elsewhere if it were reduced to a stand-alone Urgent Care Centre.

This also assumes that if patients are not admitted they were not ill enough to need an A&E in the first place. That ignores medical practice. There are cases where it is not clear, until after assessment by an Emergency Department (ED) doctor, that a person does not need to be admitted. GPs often send cases they are not sure of for ED assessment, and even if the patient is not admitted it does not mean they did not need to be seen by an ED doctor to make that judgement. This is another example of plans being drawn up by management consultants.

This assertion is grossly misleading, and not backed by any evidence. Consultants at Lewisham Emergency Department point to gross factual inaccuracies in the starting assumptions in the TSA plan, notably the drastic under-statement of the number of 'blue light' ambulances bringing the most seriously unwell patients to Lewisham's A&E each day (figures which the TSA could easily have obtained from the computerised data kept by the Department).

Lewisham ED consultants also point to the thousands of adults and children who are treated in the Rapid Assessment and Treatment Unit or the Short Stay Unit in the Children's ED – all of whom are omitted from the TSA summary and ignored as part of the caseload that would have had to be redirected to Queen Elizabeth Hospital Woolwich or elsewhere if the TSA plan had been implemented. At Lewisham Hospital the UCC works as it does *only* because it runs alongside and jointly with the A&E, and as a result has been able to deal with patients 'with problems far greater than those that can be handled in a typical UCC'. However this also means that if the A&E is closed, 'a stand-alone UCC will not be able to handle the number or acuity of patients that we presently see'.

Another important issue was staffing. The consultants pointed out that Emergency Nurse practitioners working in Lewisham's UCC 'have chosen to work in an integrated department, and there are real concerns about the retention of a very experienced workforce and future recruitment'.

The ED consultants' own estimate was that with all the factors taken into account, far from the 77 per cent figure, no more than 30 per cent of the current caseload could be safely managed in a stand-alone UCC, leaving a residual caseload too large to be dealt with in neighbouring A&E units: 'The remaining 70 per cent would have to be seen in an ED setting: there is no provision in the report as to how this could be catered for by surrounding services. Consultation with our neighbouring ED colleagues suggests that they do not have the capacity to absorb these numbers.'

Sources: (1) Trust Special Administrator, 2013. 'Securing sustainable NHS services: the Trust Special Administrator's report on South London Healthcare NHS Trust and the NHS in south east London', http://moderngov.southwark.gov.uk/documents/s35012/TSA per cent 20Final per cent20Report.pdf; and (2) Lister, J. 2013. Saving the Cancer, 'Sacrificing the Patient', http://www.healthemergency.org.uk/pdf/LondonHealthEmer gencyResponsetoTSA-Dec2012.pdf.

The College of Emergency Medicine has gone further and stated clearly that claims by Darzi, McKinsey and NHS London that 60 per cent of A&E attenders could be diverted to primary care are 'fiction'.[10] No new evidence has emerged since then to challenge this judgment, so it appears that any plans for A&E closures based on McKinsey's assumptions will be a wild gamble, based on wishful thinking rather than serious evidence-based proposals.

Why Accident and Emergency is a prime target
If the aim is to save money, why do so many reconfigurations revolve around the idea of closing an A&E? It's not because

there are big savings to be made by closing A&E. When McKinsey produced their report for NHS London in 2009,[11] outlining savings proposals, their figures showed that spending on A&E (seeing 3.8m patients) was just £300m out of £11.3bn – just 2.6 per cent of London's health budget; so even closing *all* A&E services would only make a small impact on the projected shortfall.

A&E services are incredibly 'cheap' to run, because the NHS tariff is so close to the actual cost, leaving hospital bosses no margin to cover any extra costs of agency staff, overtime and the losses incurred from the treatment of 'excess' patients above the 2009 caseload (whose care is paid at just 30 per cent of tariff costs). This means all of the financial pressure lands not on the commissioner but on the trust.

So the direct impact of closing an A&E – especially if it is replaced by alternative services in the community, or requires expansion of other A&E units in neighbouring hospitals – is in itself a marginal cost saving.* Its attraction for NHS bureaucrats is that it opens up more possibilities for cutbacks and closures in the longer term.

Almost every closure of an acute hospital since the late 1970s has begun with the closure of A&E. It marks the start of a tried and tested sequence of events, and in itself helps to create a phony 'clinical' justification for the continued process of downsizing and then closing a busy local hospital. In Chapter 6 we quoted extracts from the spoof *Briefing for Cynical Commissioning Groups* on how to 'get away with' hospital closures drawn up by campaign group Health

* Even Lord Darzi's Technical Report back in 2007 estimated the cost of an A&E-type consultation in a Polyclinic to cost £66, compared with £81 in a 'major acute or specialist' hospital (2007:23). But another NHS London sponsored study of 6 London PCTs in 2008 estimated the average cost of an A&E attendance was just £68 (PA Consulting, *Study of Unscheduled Care in 6 Primary Care Trusts Central Report*, page 27).

Emergency. It is drawn from numerous real-life consultations, and emphasises the longer-term view when it advises cynical commissioners:

> Make a strong play for your credentials as upholding 'safety' and improving patient care. Not only does this divert from what you are actually doing, but the 'safety' card can prove very handy as an excuse for the second wave of cuts that will inevitably follow on once the first wave is in place.
>
> Having reduced a site to elective services only and removed ITU (Intensive Therapy/Treatment Unit) etc., you can pick your time to argue (obviously with regret) that it can't be properly staffed, and more services need to close – perhaps 'temporarily,' and then permanently … for 'safety' reasons. This way you can get away with closures without any consultation at all.[12]

On this, the spoof accurately mirrors the way this has all been done before in real life.

- First A&E opening hours are cut back, and trauma services are removed, reducing services to out of hours medical emergencies.
- Then maternity services are cut back and then closed.
- Piece by piece the key elements that go in to making a district general hospital are hacked away, with each block removed from the package triggering others to fall – like some giant game of NHS Jenga.
- With A&E goes paediatrics, ITU, High Dependency Units and Coronary Care.
- With maternity goes women's care.
- With the loss of trauma goes orthopaedics.

- Emergency surgery is then pronounced 'unsafe' or 'unsustainable' and removed.
- Each element takes a range of supporting services with it, until the hospital is allowed to wither away, and each cutback also makes it harder to recruit medical staff and qualified nurses, opening up arguments that further cuts are required because staffing levels are inadequate.

To cap it all, trendy arguments are wheeled out by the King's Fund, McKinsey and other hired hands suggesting that new 'settings' can deliver services more efficiently and effectively than hospitals. The only snag is that these 'settings' and services exist only on paper. The vague promises of services 'closer to home' wind up with the actual closure of hospitals that local people value and depend upon, but nothing to replace them. The alternative provision of care in UCCs or GP surgeries is not a lot cheaper – and for those who have more serious health problems, nowhere near as good.

From start to finish, even though the whole cynical process is dressed up in 'clinical' arguments, the long term goal is making savings – whether from reductions in patient care, lost jobs, reduced capital costs, or even sale of 'spare' land and buildings. Another plus factor for commissioners is that a threat to an A&E will also draw almost all the attention of local public campaigning and press coverage, letting local Clinical Commissioning Group (CCGs) get on with other cuts to services such as mental health and older people's services with relatively little disruption.

Who invented these figures?

The origin of the TSA's wild guess of 77 per cent of A&E patients to be treated in a standalone Lewisham UCC or in 'the community' is a bit of a mystery. Back in 2007, Lord Darzi's report on London started the rot with the proposal (set out in the supporting McKinsey-researched Technical Paper)[13] for 50 per cent of the capital's A&E attenders to be shifted into polyclinics. This figure was then arbitrarily jacked up to 60 per cent by NHS London's Planning Guidance. The source of Darzi's original assumptions or of these revised figures has not been publicised. There has been no proper scrutiny of the evidence base or the methodology used, yet these figures have been taken as a starting point for many subsequent plans in London and elsewhere.

According to the spoof guide for *Cynical Commissioning Groups*:

> A reconfiguration needs more than just closures: it needs a ready supply of dodgy plans appearing to cut costs, improve 'productivity' and 'focus resources'. One ready source is the McKinsey report from 2009 which first mapped out ways to 'save' £20bn from the NHS – through measures including the rationing or exclusion of elective treatments including hip and knee replacements and cataract operations … or cutting doctors' consultation times…. Other old favourites include citing completely imaginary travel times to more distant hospitals.[14]

NHS London claims to have partly rested its case for reducing A&E services (and relying instead on UCCs, primary care and community services) on a report researched by PA Consulting, published in 2008. They clearly assumed nobody would check what that report really said. However the *Study of Unscheduled Care in 6 Primary Care Trusts Central Report*[15] offers little support for those seeking to inflate the numbers of minor cases in A&E. It is a detailed and nuanced 180-page study of caseload in six varied London primary care trusts, which is repeatedly at pains to stress the potential for bias in its findings and the complexity of the issues it is analysing. It makes much more limited claims than NHS London on the level of 'inappropriate' attendances at A&E.

Another report, *Primary Care and Emergency Departments* commissioned from the Primary Care Foundation by the Department of Health in 2010, questioned the assumptions on how many A&E attenders could be adequately treated in a primary care setting.[16] The Department of Health's specific brief was to 'provide a viable estimate of the number of patients who attend emergency department with conditions that could be dealt with elsewhere in primary care'.[16] Yet even from this starting point the researchers found that relatively few patients attending hospital Accident and Emergency departments could be classified as needing only primary care – suggesting that NHS London had drastically overstated the case for shifting work out of hospital A&E. The 102-page report specifically took issue with 'widespread assumptions that up to 60 per cent of patients could be diverted to GPs or primary care nurses', and argued that the real figure is as low as 10-30 per cent.[17]

Significantly the extensive study of patients in actual A&E departments also found no evidence that providing primary care in Emergency Departments 'could tackle rising costs or help to avoid unnecessary admissions'. The authors of the report also question the financial case for diverting patients from A&E, arguing that 'cost benefits may exist, but the evidence is weak.'[18]

Among Health Emergency's spoof suggestions, all drawn from real life 'consultations', is the advice to:

Ignore any questions on embarrassing figures and issues that might discredit your argument – such as figures showing the continued rise in emergency admissions and referrals, the pressure on hospital beds, the spiralling workload on over-stressed staff, the levels of deprivation and other specific needs of a local population, etc.

Just ignore them. Ministers won't hear them, and will back you anyway.

The Trust Special Administrator followed this approach to insist that 77 per cent of patients in Lewisham could be handled through a free-standing UCC or in community based services. This same misleading claim helped to secure the plan a spurious clean bill of health in the *Health Equalities Impact Assessment* drawn up for the TSA by Deloitte. After reluctantly admitting that Lewisham's population suffers high levels of deprivation, and that this deprived population would suffer if journey times to access treatment were increased. Deloitte countered this by using the spurious 77 per cent figure:

As Lewisham has a number of deprived wards, this impact will need to be considered in greater detail. However it is estimated that between 70 per cent and 80 per cent of patients currently receiving treatment at University Hospital Lewisham (UHL) A&E could be treated at its urgent care centre, potentially abating the scale of this impact.[19]

Since clinicians' views and evidence are so blatantly disregarded in this plan to downgrade a busy A&E department (and similar plans elsewhere), what grounds are there for believing the claim that such plans are 'clinically led' rather than driven by concerns over balance sheets?

Reliance on abstractions and assertions

In Bedfordshire, too, similar arguments have been wheeled out by a Clinical Commissioning Group seeking to drive a rationalisation of services in Bedford and Milton Keynes. Their plans,[20] which were contested by a strong local campaign, have since been shelved until after the election, but not yet abandoned. They looked to scale down hospital care in one trust or both – suggesting that local people might as readily use other 'nearby' hospitals – all of them between 20 and 50 miles away.

The proposals were backed up by a series of abstract assertions – for example that 20 per cent of people who go to a GP turn out to have 'self-treatable minor ailments' – without explaining how people are supposed to diagnose this themselves, and distinguish their 'minor ailments' from early symptoms of more serious problems. Nor do they show how this questionable statistic relates to their plans to scale down hospital services.

Bedfordshire health chiefs also argue that 50 per cent of 999 ambulance calls 'could be managed at the scene'. This assumes that sufficient properly trained and equipped paramedics have the time and facilities to do so. However there is no explanation of why they don't do this now, or what proportion of cases are already managed at the scene.

Apparently a million emergency hospital admissions were 'considered avoidable' by somebody or other in 2012-13.

Again no explanation is offered on where these figures came from, how they were derived, or how this claim squares with other very different findings. What alternative services outside hospital would need to be in place to avoid these emergency admissions?

In a ludicrous contradiction, the same set of figures, also quoted by Bedfordshire and Milton Keynes health managers, shows that just 4 per cent (960,000) of the 24 million calls to NHS 111 emergency lines could be resolved on the phone. It seems that not all callers are just timewasters after all.

Clinical – or cynical?

We don't have to look very far to find the financial pressures behind the reconfiguration plans. NHS London's *Integrated Strategic Plan 2010-15,* published in January 2010, just months before the coalition government took office, warned[21] that urgent action was needed to bridge a potential 'funding shortfall of between £3.8bn and £5.1bn per year in the capital on a recurrent basis' by 2016. These figures are strikingly similar to the projections of NHS England's London region looking forward from 2013. This is clearly the starting point for the subsequent plans for huge cost savings – including reconfiguration. These savings were part of a massive programme of cuts throughout England: the *Health Service Journal* estimated the total of hospital trusts' planned 'cash savings' for 2012-13 at £2.35bn.[22]

In north-west London, too, it's clear that the unspoken driver is in fact the prospect of a £1bn cash gap between resources and local need for health care. To bridge at least some of this gap the PCTs in the eight boroughs of north-west London organised together as 'NHS North West London' (NHSNWL) in 2010-11, and drew up plans to slash £314m from north-west London hospital budgets over three years, as well as cutting £297m from health commissioning budgets.[23]

The CCGs, which have taken over the plans from their predecessor the primary care trusts (PCTs), also want to open up the health budgets of north-west London to 'Any Qualified Provider', to create the kind of competitive market in health care outlined in the Health and Social Care Act. To do this means further undermining the financial viability of established NHS providers, and reducing their capacity. And new providers could only help CCGs save money while also pocketing a profit if they are encouraged to compete on price, and encouraged to offer a 'cheap and cheerful' downgraded service with reduced reliance on better qualified staff.

So however much the plans are said to be the work of 'clinicians', and are presented as improvements under the heading *Shaping a Healthier Future*,[24] in fact they are driven first and foremost by financial concerns – and the attempt to curb spending.

Much more recently, CCGs in the five counties of what was formerly the East Midland Strategic Health Authority have identified a combined savings target for health and social care over the next five years of more than £1bn – almost 20 per cent of the current budget – while local trusts already faced deficits of almost £150m in 2014-15. As the pressure mounts for cuts and closures – even contemplating reducing sprawling Lincolnshire with its scattered population and inadequate road network to just a single A&E – pressures and demands on frontline services continue to increase, and the numbers of more vulnerable older people are growing even faster than the general population.[25]

From moratorium to more closures

In the summer of 2010, just weeks after the election in which he and David Cameron had made so many promises, Andrew Lansley travelled to the threatened A&E at Chase Farm Hospital in Enfield to make his announcement of a 'moratorium' on closures of A&E and maternity units. He pledged to halt the 'top-down process that forces closure', but made it clear he offered a stay of execution rather than a full reprieve. He refused to guarantee the A&E department would be saved, or say how long the moratorium on cuts would last. He told reporters: 'I can't rule out change, I can't rule out A&E closures. But we will stop forced closures. We will take away all decisions not clinically based, which don't conform to patients' needs.'

Well at least the first two statements were correct. Closures of local services including A&E were by no means ruled out – as long as they could be claimed somehow to comply with Lansley's minimal new preconditions.

The management were never fooled, and the promise didn't last too long. Barely was the ink dry on Lansley's authorisation of the moratorium before it was clear that the delay would be just a couple of months across the summer of 2010.

So while the hotly contested closure of Chase Farm's A&E was postponed for a while (although it eventually closed its doors at the end of 2013) in south-east London, Queen Mary's Hospital, Sidcup, whose A&E and other services were threatened as part of a desperate plan to restore financial viability to the South London Hospitals Trust, was the first of many that were still set to lose most of their services.

This was despite opportunist claims by the local Tory candidate, James Brokenshire, made just before the election to have secured a pledge from Lansley that St Mary's would be reprieved. The claims were soon discredited. By the autumn of 2010 key services were already closing down, in the beginnings of a process that has now left almost no services on the site.

False assumptions

A similar fate would have befallen King George's Hospital in Ilford if the assumptions on which the closure was supposed to be manageable had not been so disastrously and visibly wide of the mark. King George's has for years been part of the Barking, Havering & Redbridge NHS trust, which since 2006 has been struggling unsuccessfully to cover the inflated costs of payments on its PFI-funded £226m Queen's Hospital in Romford.* King George's sits on a site two thirds of which could be sold off. This hospital has no PFI bills attached; closing it has always been above all about saving money and relieving the financial distress of its parent trust.

But Queen's Hospital (as critics had warned) had been built with too few beds, and the Trust has been in such dire financial straits that it was unable even to afford the staff to make use of the whole of the costly new building, leaving a whole floor closed at considerable expense, while the remaining beds ran at full tilt. The only factor saving the Trust from total meltdown was the availability of beds at King George's – beds that would be axed if the plan to shut down most of the busy 20-year old hospital, bulldoze two thirds of the site and sell off the land were carried through. The closure has been postponed to 2015, but still no real plans are in place for what would happen to the patients displaced

* According to official Treasury figures, the Trust has so far paid £387m for the hospital, but still has another £1.8bn to pay – costing a hefty 9.7 times the initial capital investment.

when it goes.

Of course, none of the closure plans in London or elsewhere are ever presented as closures. Instead, they are painted up as 'reconfigurations' to centralise services in other hospitals, where teams of eager consultants will toil seven days a week, 24 hours a day. A diplomatic silence always obscures the fact that few of these new 'centres' would in reality have any of the investment in resources and extra beds they would need to deal with the additional caseload if another local hospital was closed.

The spoof *Briefing for Cynical Commissioning Groups* on 'how to get away with it' emphasises the need to give the impression that the axed services would be replaced by something different but better:

> Imply – or even promise – you will replace hospital care with a range of services 'closer to patients' homes' or 'in the community'. Never mind the fact you're closing the nearest hospital, or that there is no evidence these services can replace A&E – or that there's no money to pay for them.[26]

In fact, hardly any of the fabled community-based or primary care 'alternative settings' for care actually exist. Time and again a close reading of strategic plans for reconfiguration reveals the same sad story of deception: there are no staff, no premises, no plan, no money and really no political will to establish these services – which may well prove more expensive and less efficient than the hospitals they are supposed to replace. Local GPs, mostly keeping their heads down and ignoring the reconfiguration process, hoping that the worst won't happen, are in many cases already struggling, and their services in some cases are less than consistently good. There is little chance that they could absorb the vast increase in workload that the planners are proposing to dump onto them with the closure of hospitals.

The spoof *Briefing* urges CCGs:

Wherever possible avoid offering any concrete plans for alternative services. You are trying to save money, not spend it. Your only concrete plans, with timescales for implementation should be your cuts and closures. Remember it's always easier not to make a promise than to break one.

Many areas are struggling to recruit and retain GPs – and the shortage of these and other crucial staff, such as district nurses, seems set to worsen. It's all a big exercise in deception – in some cases the self-deception of well-meaning bureaucrats accepting some spurious 'evidence' of policies they are being pressed to implement, and hoping it will all turn out for the best. In other cases there is more cynical deception in the management offices or consultancy firms where the spurious figures and claims originate. Whatever the motivation, the consequences of half-baked plans are the same: gaps in care, failing services and patients put at risk.

The *Francis Report* in February 2013,[27] learning one of the key lessons from the Mid Staffordshire Hospitals debacle, spelled out the duty of directors and senior managers to point out when resources are inadequate to deliver safe and satisfactory services, rather than muddle on inflicting cuts which make it impossible for professional staff to do their jobs properly. This duty should apply with equal force to commissioners who find themselves driven towards policies by financial constraints. Sadly too many of them seem to feel they can simply pass their problems on to the frontline providers, who have no line of escape, and who wind up carrying the can when staff shortages or delays in treatment result in harm to patients.

Are alternatives any cheaper? Do they even work?

NHS London's *Integrated Strategic Plan* argued that five interventions could between them save up to £3.1bn.[28] Many of these consist of delivering less care, or seeking to bury the identifiable costs of delivering hospital services in a general heading of community or primary care.

The proposed interventions were:

- Reducing the cost of services delivered in the community.
- Providing more care in the community and less in hospitals.
- Stopping clinical interventions which NHS London argues 'have little or no benefit to those receiving them' – including 'some joint replacements' (although no more detail is offered).
- Proactive care for people with long-term conditions, reducing the need for hospital admissions.
- Prevention to reduce the risk of ill-health.*

In practice the evidence for cost savings from developing GP and community out of hospital initiatives is very limited. Research published in 2012 surveying all out of hospital initiatives failed to demonstrate savings.[29]

* Which some PCTs and now CCGs, together with NHS England's chief executive Simon Stevens seem to have rather naively interpreted as enabling almost instant results from long-term preventive policies.

Also in 2012 an analytical paper in the *BMJ* by Professor Martin Roland and Gary Abel[30] questioned the received wisdom that hospital admissions could be reduced and costs cut by improving primary care interventions, especially those aimed at high risk patients (whose chronic health problems often lead to them being pejoratively dismissed by NHS bureaucrats as 'frequent flyers'). Among the bevy of myths dispelled by this study is the illusion that high risk patients account for most admissions, or that case management of such patients could save money:

[M]ost admissions come from low risk patients, and the greatest effect on admissions will be made by reducing risk factors in the whole population....

... even with the high risk group, the numbers start to cause a problem for any form of case management intervention – 5 per cent of an average general practitioner's list is 85 patients. To manage this caseload would require 1 to 1.5 case managers per GP. This would require a huge investment of NHS resources in an intervention for which there is no strong evidence that it reduces emergency admissions.

Roland also points out the difficulties of assessing the effectiveness of those interventions that have taken place because of fluctuations in numbers of admissions even among those at high risk. Some of the interventions that have been piloted, providing case management for high risk groups of patients, have proved not only ineffective, but to result in increased numbers of emergency admissions – possibly because the increased level of care resulted in additional problems being identified. Indeed three trials of interventions have had to be abandoned because of increased deaths among the patients involved. Roland warns that an additional unintended negative consequence could result from GPs feeling under 'excessive' pressure not to refer sick patients to hospital. And Roland criticises the failure of many plans aimed at reducing hospital admissions to consider the role of secondary care, and improved collaboration between GPs and hospital colleagues.

Promising to locate more and more services in smaller, community settings 'closer to home' makes good sound-bites, especially when this is being used as a smokescreen to divert attention from the closure of convenient nearby hospitals, requiring many patients with more serious problems to travel even further from home. But there are real questions to be asked about the costs and efficiencies involved, and availability of essential, but sometimes scarce professional staff. Most would agree that neighbourhood access to MRI scanning, for example, or proton beam therapy makes little sense. These resources need to be shared across much wider populations to ensure that they are adequately used and staffed by appropriately skilled staff.

For similar reasons there were questions over the viability of including X-ray imaging in Lord Darzi's planned polyclinics, which would raise the need for larger buildings, with lead-lined rooms and costly equipment, and for radiographers and radiologists who are in short supply. Likewise it's not clear why NHS England CEO Simon Stevens' idea of GP practices employing hospital consultants makes any financial or organisational sense.[31] Highly specialist consultants would be obliged to spend time dealing with much smaller hyper-local lists of patients rather than being based together with other consultants (and training junior doctors) in hospitals covering larger populations, developing multi-disciplinary teams.

Is it a good use of the time of highly skilled professional staff for them to be travelling around from one GP practice or relatively small health centre to another to see small groups of patients, rather than working continuously from a central base – and one that already exists, and is known to patients? How does it make financial sense to equip small-scale local health centres and GP surgeries with the costly equipment needed for even the most basic consultations, when it would be used only occasionally?

There seems to be a contradiction between wanting to save money and work more productively on the one hand, and the consumerist idea of specialists running round to deal with individuals and small groups of patients on the other. Given the economic constraints that hang over the NHS and the absence of the long-promised new expansion of community-based services, it seems the utmost folly to move to a less efficient, more fragmented system that could cost more without enhancing the quality of patient care – at the same time annoying whole communities whose hospitals and local services could be put at risk in the process.

Conclusions

This chapter has referred to evidence, academic research conducted for the NHS, and to practical examples to underline the fact that the case for hospital (and in particular A&E) closures has not been made. Instead of evidence, commissioners and hard-pressed hospital trusts have time and again relied on assumptions about care in the community which are either unproven, or worse, downright wrong. They have made selective and inappropriate use of statistics, and drawn inappropriate conclusions from the experience of well-resourced and widely accepted centralisation of specialised stroke and trauma services – in the hope of persuading local people to accept unpalatable loss of local access to emergency services. In misleading strategic documents and Business Cases they have repeatedly tried to pass off generic arguments for reconfiguration as tailored to 'local' circumstances, and put forward at best vague future aspirations to expand community and primary health services as sufficient grounds for short-term closure and downgrading of actual services.

This implausible line of argument to justify closures of A&E has been immediately and crushingly refuted. We noted in Chapter 6 the collapse in A&E performance that immediately followed from the closure of two A&E units in north-west London, despite repeated promises that alternative services would be put in place beforehand.

The only serious ministerial approach to the issue of reconfiguration came from Lord Darzi while he was still a Labour minister. His five pledges, designed to reassure concerned communities faced with reconfiguration of local services, amount to the direct opposite of the way reconfiguration, set out in his 2008 *Next Stage Review*,[32] has been approached, before and since.

- Change will always be to the benefit of patients.
- Change will be clinically driven.
- All change will be locally-led.
- You will be involved.
- You will see the difference first.*

* One wag suggested that the pledges would better reflect the reality of reconfiguration if the word 'not' were to be inserted in each pledge.

David Cameron's Tory party contested the last election opposing financially-driven closures, but almost immediately changed tack once in office, and through its planned ten-year freeze on real terms spending is forcing the pace in local cuts and closures, despite a total failure to win public consent. Where will the next government stand? Will they apply the Darzi pledges? Will evidence and good sense win out? Or will the myths and deceptions continue to prevail?

11

What they don't want us to know

The NHS is a huge and complex organisation with a UK budget of over £120bn. It employs 1.7 million people and only the Chinese People's Liberation Army, Walmart and the Indian Railways directly employ more people. It is the most popular institution in the country and voters are attached to it for sentimental as well as sound practical reasons. No government can afford to be judged to have made a mess of it let alone begun a relentless privatisation programme that no one voted for or wanted. No politician wants to be associated with a downturn in its fortunes.

But since the coalition came into power, the passing of their Health and Social Care Act and the imposition of massive financial cuts have had a very damaging effect on the NHS. Their legislation has also opened up opportunities for big profits to be made and political favours to be called in. The resulting threats to the NHS, along with rumours of financial conflicts of interest, have required some nifty public relations footwork by the coalition government. It really does not suit them for the voters to know the truth about what is being done to the NHS, by whom, and how much money they are making out of it.

What the Tories really think about the NHS
The Tories have never been honest about their real intentions for the NHS, but in January 2011 former contender for the Tory leadership Michael Portillo made a startling admission

to the BBC's Andrew Neil. He let slip that in the run-up to the 2010 general election the Tories had not been entirely honest about their intentions for the NHS: 'They did not believe they could win an election if they told you what they were going to do because people are so wedded to the NHS.'[1]

Portillo was of course alluding to the Health and Social Care Bill – the most controversial piece of NHS legislation in recent generations. The Conservative manifesto and indeed even the coalition agreement made no mention of the assault on the NHS that had been planned for many years by Tory politicians.* But anyone who had been paying attention should not have been surprised when a massive piece of privatising legislation appeared within weeks of the 2010 Tory-led coalition taking power. They had already heard Oliver Letwin, the Tory policy guru, claim there would be no NHS within five years of a Tory government,[2] and had read his book *Privatising the World* (see Chapter 9). However abhorrent Letwin's sentiments they did at least have the virtue of being honest.

The same could not be said of David Cameron's lies before the 2010 election. In a speech at the Royal College of Pathologists on 2 November 2009, Cameron promised an end to further 're-disorganisations' of the NHS and a steady ship after a Tory victory: 'With the Conservatives there will be no more of the tiresome, meddlesome, top-down restructures that have dominated the last decade of the NHS.' He repeated the promise, and was even captured for posterity on YouTube at a Royal College of Nursing congress, basking in prolonged applause from the audience when he told them:

* *The Plot against the NHS* (Leys and Player) is an essential read for anyone who wants to know more about the relentless political manoeuvring against the NHS.

First I want to tell you what we're not going to do. There will be no more of those pointless re-organisations that aim for change but instead bring chaos. Too often ministers have rearranged the NHS as if they were shuffling a deck of cards and not the nation's largest employer … The recent history of the NHS reads like a wretched bowl of alphabeti spaghetti and it has got to stop.[3]

His reception might have been less enthusiastic if he had told the cheering nurses that within two years thousands of their members would have lost their jobs while he presided over the biggest ever reorganisation of the NHS. Little wonder that each year politicians come out as the least trusted profession.[4]

The coalition certainly didn't want the public to know the purpose behind the HSC Act, but others were more forthright. Kingsley Manning, business development director at Tribal in 2010, welcomed the proposed legislation saying it 'could lead to the denationalization of health care services in England'.[5] He went on to be appointed Chair of the Health and Social Care Information Centre.

Cui bono – who stood to profit?

The HSC Act was a stark betrayal of Cameron's clear promise that he would not reorganise the NHS but, worse than that, it was a betrayal of the NHS itself. Messing with the NHS and failing goes against all political advice, but those who wondered why the Tories would take such a risk with the nation's favourite institution didn't have to look very far. No further indeed than the financial interests of their MPs and peers and the pressures from donors and lobbying organisations.

In 2012 the website 'socialinvestigations'[6] published a compilation of the financial and vested interests of those who voted on the HSCB (updated in 2013). They were unapologetic about the long list of over 200 parliamentarians who had voted and who had present or recent past connections with companies involved in private health care, seeing it as a reflection of the 'tragic reality' of current politics. They pointed out what should be obvious even to an ethics class of five year olds – that having a Register of Members' Financial Interests doesn't excuse parliamentarians' interests, but merely highlights why they should not have been allowed to vote on important legislation from which they stood to profit.

It is worth listing some of its findings:

- Some 225 parliamentarians had recent or current financial interests in private health care.
- 145 peers had recent or present financial connections to companies or individuals involved in health care.
- One in four Conservative peers had recent or present financial connections to companies or individuals involved in health care.
- One in six Labour peers have recent or present financial connections to companies or individuals involved in health care.

Although 78 per cent of the MPs listed were Tory it became apparent that the issue was a cross-party one, although (with the notable exception of former health minister Lord Warner), Labour parliamentarians opposed the health reforms. The conflicts of interest they exposed constitute a running sore in a country with pretensions to democracy.

The investigation revealed a tangled web of offshore

companies, donations, consultancies, directorships and shares held in companies likely to profit from the legislation's privatisation agenda. 'Socialinvestigations' asked whether these people were public or corporate servants, a question which the reader will not find hard to answer after they have read their report – highly recommended but not for the squeamish or faint hearted.[7] Particularly difficult to stomach are the excerpts from the speeches of those with direct financial conflicts of interest. 'Extraordinarily' warm welcomes were extended to the Bill along with calls for more use of management consultants and the 'independent' sector. Apart from the light it sheds on MPs extra-curricular activities, the whole report stands on its own as a damning indictment of the House of Lords, and the cat's cradle of political and financial influence wielded by unelected peers.

Meanwhile Tory party donors have done nicely under the new regime. In 2013 the coalition government awarded a controversial contract to treat brain tumours to Hospital Corporation of America (HCA), just days before responsibility for such contracts passed to NHS England. HCA were already at the centre of a scandal about overcharging the NHS by millions of pounds, and had a record of paying over $1bn in fines in the US for mis-selling health care, but regardless of their history the highly specialised work was taken away from University College Hospital (UCH) and given to HCA and another private company. Patients who were already being treated at UCH were told to move to the private company as their treatment at UCH would no longer be funded. An investigation by *The Mirror* revealed that HCA was a Tory party donor, and had given them 'at least' £17,000 since the election.[8]

Lord Popat is a Ugandan born British Asian businessman

who has donated over £320,000 to the Conservative party and was subsequently made a peer in July 2010. He supported and voted for the Health and Social Care Act and was made a Government Whip and Minister of the Crown in 2013. He founded the company TLC which owns a string of care homes offering services to the NHS, and gave the Tories £25,000 just a week after they unveiled their healthcare reforms. Unite the Union discovered Lord Popat's wife now owns the company which has won contracts worth £4.43m since the HSC Act was passed in 2012.[9]

In October 2014 *The Guardian* published an article (based on a Unite report) about links between Tory MPs and NHS contracts awarded to the private sector. Private companies with financial links to 24 Tory MPs and peers had won NHS contracts worth £1.5bn under the new legislation. A Conservative spokesman was suitably outraged at the implication and denied any wrongdoing: 'Any suggestion of impropriety is malicious and defamatory and will be treated as such.'[10]

Len McCluskey of Unite was not deterred: 'How can we be in a situation where dozens of [Cameron's] MPs voted for the sell-off act and had links to private healthcare companies, knowing this would open up new opportunities for the companies that pay them?'[11]

It is worth looking at a few individuals who distinguished themselves during this period

Andrew Lansley

Andrew Lansley was the architect and driver of the HSC Act, labelled by the *BMJ* 'Lansley's monster'. In November 2009 John Nash, chairman of Care UK, donated £21,000 to Lansley's private office.[12] At that stage Care UK had contracts worth £400 million derived from the NHS – 96 per cent of their total income. An article in *The Telegraph* noted that Mr Nash, a private equity tycoon, stood to be one of the biggest beneficiaries of Conservative policies to increase the use of private healthcare providers.

Lansley denied that the £21,000 donation would have swayed him or the party in any way whatsoever, and the usual spokesperson was wheeled out to say that 'donations from private individuals in no way influence policy making decisions'. Clearly believing otherwise, John Nash and his wife donated almost £300,000 to the Conservative party. In January 2013 Nash was rewarded with a life peerage – Baron Nash, of Ewelme in the County of Oxfordshire – and was subsequently made Parliamentary Under-Secretary of State for Schools in the Cameron coalition government – an appropriate appointment for an enthusiastic sponsor of the loathed academy programme.[13]

Lord Warner

On the other side of the House on the Labour benches sits Lord Warner (although after the passage of the HSC Act many wondered if that was quite where he belonged). Warner was made a life peer by Tony Blair in 1998, since when he has been, among other things, Minister of State in the Department of Health from 2005 to 2007. Of more than passing interest is that he also sits on the advisory board of Reform – a right-wing 'think tank' funded to the tune of around £1m by private companies that stand to benefit financially from a privatised NHS.[14]

Warner had a reputation as a Blairite on the right of the Labour Party, and true to his colours he announced in April 2013 that he would break ranks and vote with the coalition on section 75, a crucial piece of NHS legislation. Section 75 regulations were designed to push CCGs down the route of tendering out NHS services, making tendering in effect compulsory. Section 75 thus meant private companies would have many more opportunities to bid for high value NHS contracts in the future.

Lord Warner denied that the regulations would mean compulsory competitive tendering in the NHS and claimed disingenuously to be 'voting in the best interests of NHS patients'.[15] Some felt his connections with private sector health care might have played a part in his decision to defy a three line whip, and one blogger simply stated that Warner stood to make 'shedloads of money' out of NHS privatisation and congratulated the peer on his chutzpah in not apparently caring whether anyone made the connection.[16]

Some saw Warner's vote as an act of betrayal and there were calls for him to resign from the Labour Party and stick with Reform as his lobbying group of choice. Lord Philip Hunt (Shadow Deputy Leader of the House of Lords and spokesman on health) had worked hard to mobilise opposition to section 75 and tweeted on 24 April 2013: 'Very disappointed with outcome of Lords vote on section 75 competition regulations. But a massive thanks to all who have campaigned on this.' One of the authors, John Lister, tweeted back: 'What will Labour do about Lord Warner who declared personal interests and then broke with the Labour whip to support the government.' The answer was they would do nothing – Lord Warner remains on the Labour benches, having committed this act of betrayal and helped consign the English NHS to a further expansion of privatisation.

In order not to disappoint his critics Lord Warner was back in the headlines again in March 2014. On this occasion he wrote a pamphlet for Reform, recommending charging for NHS services, an issue that for most is an NHS red line and not to be crossed. In a *Guardian* article he claimed without evidence that the NHS was poor value for money[17] and called for a £10 a month NHS membership fee.[18] Reform advocate patient charges,[19] and given Lord Warner's role as an adviser to them it came as no surprise that he was waving their flag, but he attracted the anger of his Parliamentary colleagues. Labour health spokesman Jamie Reed MP disavowed Warner's recommendations: 'This is not something Labour would ever consider ... a Labour government will repeal David Cameron's NHS changes that put private profit before patient care.'[20]

Alan Milburn

Alan Milburn's name and reputation are well known in the field of health care. He went from firebrand opposition spokesman putting the Major government on the spot, to marketising health secretary, and then on to a directorship in private health (now coupled with a role advising David Cameron's government on social mobility). Milburn was MP for Darlington from 1992-2010 and his role has been well documented elsewhere as the architect of the New Labour love affair with the private sector in health care, much of which was set out in the 2000 NHS Plan. It was Milburn (interestingly with Simon Stevens – now head of NHS England – at his side) who signed the concordat with the private health industry in 2000 that opened up NHS services in England to the private sector,[21] amongst other things sending NHS elective patients for treatment (during winter peaks) in private hospitals at much higher cost. Milburn also pushed through many of the PFI deals which are still crippling NHS hospitals to this day, and he was also the inspiration behind turning hospitals into businesses and pitching them against each other – the foundation trust initiative.

The actions of New Labour ministers such as Milburn allowed the Tories to claim with some justification that with the HSC Act they were only carrying on with what Labour had started. In 2012, a Downing Street source was quoted as saying that Lansley should be taken out and shot for the mess he had made of the health reforms, and had to deny the rumour that Milburn could be given a peerage and asked to return to his old job to replace Lansley and steer the troubled reforms through parliament.[22]

Milburn went on to become a consultant to Bridgepoint, a venture capital firm heavily involved in financing healthcare firms moving into the NHS, including Alliance Medical, Match Group, Medica and Care UK.[23] In 2013 Milburn was appointed by PriceWaterhouseCoopers (PwC), the world's largest accountancy and consultancy firm, to head up a board overseeing its healthcare practice. Milburn commented: 'The health industry in the UK offers strong opportunities for growth in the wider economy and for PwC. My aim is to bring together a panel of industry experts to help catalyse change across the health sector and to help PwC grow its presence in the health market.'[24]

The revolving door

Alan Milburn graduated from being a health minister pushing NHS privatisation to jobs in the same private sector which benefited from his policies. His story exemplifies the 'revolving door' between the public and private worlds which has spun faster and faster of late, seeing politicians and civil servants moving into lucrative posts in what Milburn tellingly calls 'the health industry' and the 'health market'. Former health ministers seem to be particularly liable to go through the door into the private sector, using contacts they made while public servants to further their private interest. The following examples are taken from the Alliance for Lobbying Transparency web site:

- Tony Newton, now Lord Newton of Braintree, a former Tory health minister in the '80s, now a paid adviser to Oasis Healthcare.
- Virginia Bottomley, ex-secretary of state for health in the early '90s, is a director of BUPA.
- Baroness Julia Cumberlege, ex-health minister in the '90s, now runs her own consultancy advising, among others, the pharmaceutical industry.
- John Bowis, another former Tory health minister, now chair of the Health Advisory Board of pharma giant GSK, and an advisor to lobby firm Hanover.
- Tom Sackville, ex-Tory health minister from the '90s, today heads up the International Federation of Health Plans, which represents one hundred private health insurance companies. Also chair of the pro-market think tank 2020health.
- Melanie Johnson, ex-public health minister became an advisor to the Association of the British Pharmaceutical

Industry.

- Patricia Hewitt, former Labour health secretary who had previously worked for Anderson Consulting (now Accenture), took a couple of paid jobs in private health care, one with Alliance Boots, another with an investment firm Cinven, which specialises in buy-outs in the healthcare industry.
- Lord Warner, former Labour health minister, took up a position with Apax Partners, one of the leading private equity investors in health care.
- Lord Darzi, another Labour ex-health minister, now an advisor to giant GE Healthcare.[25]

In 2012 *The Guardian* reported that Sean Worth, Cameron's advisor on NHS privatisation, had moved to a group whose clients included a number of firms involved in selling services to the NHS. Peter Campbell, another special advisor in No. 10, moved to the Business Services Association which represents outsourcing companies including those interested in health. The Advisory Committee on Business Appointments which decides whether top civil servants can move to the private sector, reported that 213 senior civil servants moved from government into the private health sector between 1996 and 2011.[26]

There is of course traffic in the opposite direction, albeit usually temporary, as those with their feet firmly in the private sector embed themselves in the NHS to advise ministers and influence policy. At one stage the NHS Commercial Directorate (set up as early as 2003 to help introduce private providers into the NHS) contained 190 staff, 182 of whom were 'interims' i.e. people recruited on short-term contracts from the private sector (at a daily cost to the NHS of £1000-£2000 each).[27] In 2011 the DoH sued the head of the Directorate, Ken Anderson, for accepting gifts, and the case was subsequently settled out of court.[28]

Others migrate comfortably back and forth between the two sectors. Simon Stevens was policy advisor to two health secretaries, Frank Dobson and Alan Milburn, and then to Tony Blair himself. He then moved into the private sector, ending up as executive vice-president of UnitedHealth group, one of the biggest US multinationals.

In 2003 he told a US conference 'the era of English exceptionalism in healthcare is over'. He pointed out the similarity between UK trusts now set up to 'buy' health from doctors and hospitals, and US 'managed care' organisations such as UnitedHealth. 'Indeed' he said, 'pilot programmes are now testing the partnering of US managed care plans with primary care trusts.'

He promoted choice: 'Freestanding surgical centres run by international private operators ... are a first step. Private diagnostics and primary out-of-hours services are next.'[29]

Since April 2014 he has been back in the UK as CEO of NHS England.* On the first day of his new job he laid out his stall and upset many by praising the innovation value of new providers (i.e. the private sector) in the provision of health services.[30] He has subsequently produced a heavyweight report (*The NHS Five Year Forward View*) looking at how to fund the NHS without so much as a suggestion that the English NHS market might be unnecessary and expensive or that doing away with it could save billions of pounds a year.

---

* One person who had been expected to apply for Stevens' new job at NHS England was the former NHS Director General of Commissioning Mark Britnell, who quit his senior post in 2009 to become a partner and Head of Healthcare in Europe & UK for KPMG.

Don't mention the NHS

Lynton Crosby is an Australian political strategist, described as 'master of the dark political arts' and the 'wizard of Oz'. He masterminded successful election victories in Australia and the Tories 2005 election campaign and in November 2012 was brought back as campaign consultant to the Conservative Party for the 2015 General Election.

Crosby has close links to the tobacco industry, having been hired by Philip Morris International, makers of Marlboro cigarettes.[31] There were accusations that just before his appointment Crosby lobbied a minister against the introduction of plain packaging for cigarettes (a policy felt by public health experts to significantly reduce the attractiveness of cigarettes to younger smokers and those being tempted to smoke for the first time). Crosby denied the accusations despite an e-mail trail, but the government postponed its plans to introduce plain packaging until early 2015.

As negative headlines about the NHS appeared with monotonous regularity in 2014 Cameron must have rued both his slovenly attitude to Lansley's flawed legislation and his earlier claims that his priorities could be summed up in three letters: NHS. By June 2014, with the NHS moving up into second position among voters' concerns, the *New Statesman* reported that Crosby had advised Cameron and the party not to mention the NHS.[32] As a result of the toxic 'reforms' and swingeing cuts it had become a vote loser for them and Crosby must have calculated that a period of silence was the best they could do.

Presumably on Crosby's advice there was no mention of Cameron's erstwhile top priority in that year's Queen's speech. In his 2014 pre-election conference speech Cameron made no attempt to address the NHS and its problems but instead disgracefully used his personal family tragedy to suggest that he was beyond suspicion when it came to the NHS. In a faux rage he demanded 'How dare [Labour] suggest I would ever put it at risk? How dare they frighten those who rely on the NHS?' It was a cheap shot but the media let it go unchallenged, as with so many of his other dubious assertions. Round One to Crosby.

Care.data

In 2003 the Department of Health asked computer firms to design a system that would automatically upload patients' confidential GP medical records to a centrally held database, the 'Summary Care Record' (SCR). This would happen regardless of whether patients wanted their data shared in this way. The taxpayer-funded multi-billion-pound NHS project soon ran into trouble and in 2006 Accenture (the world's largest management consultancy firm) pulled out of contracts worth £2bn.[33]

They could have been forced to pay penalties of up to £1bn but the then director general of NHS IT, Richard Granger, decided to charge Accenture just a trifling £63m.[34] Accenture must have been pleased with their 'windfall' of over £900m and it is interesting to note in passing that prior to Richard Granger working for the NHS his previous role was with Andersen Consulting, which changed its name to Accenture in 2001.*

* He was was paid £285,000 a year by the NHS in 2006 – the highest paid civil servant in the country at that time. Even his mother was shocked when she heard of his new role. 'I can't believe that my son is running the IT modernisation programme for the whole of the NHS' she is quoted as saying, having told a newspaper he failed his computer studies course when he was at Bristol University. Mrs Granger was at that time campaigning to save services in her local hospital in Halifax and went on to say 'some of the money going into Connecting for Health could be saving my local services' (http://www.theguardian.com/society/2006/nov/12/epublic.technology).

The project, Connecting for Health, was initially supp-osed to cost the taxpayer £2.3bn but in the end it cost an estimated £12.4bn (with some putting the overall cost at nearer a staggering £30bn).[35] The National Audit Office was highly critical, stating that '… it was not demonstrated that the financial values of the benefits exceeds the cost of the programme'.[36]

The resulting loss of confidence by the public and medical professions in NHS IT led the new coalition government in 2010/11 to come up with a different idea for sharing medical records – care.data. The coalition hid the new quango (the Health and Social Care Information Centre – HSCIC), which would oversee usage of confidential patient data, deep in the fiendishly complex Health and Social Care Bill.[37] The new project would allow confidential medical information to be shared and initially ministers announced that once again 'there would be no opportunity to opt out' for patients – a truly astonishing proposition.[38]

Patients trust that the information they impart to their GPs will be treated as confidential, not shared with others outside the NHS and not used for purposes other than direct patient care. This forms the basis of the sacrosanct doctor/patient relationship and if patients lose trust in data confidentiality there is the risk that they will not be open with doctors which could in turn have an effect on the care they receive. In a short period of time the politicians and HSCIC moved to destroy that trust.

Jeremy Hunt (by then Secretary of State for Health after Lansley had been demoted to the Leader of the House) stated there was 'enormous potential' for care.data to improve patient care. Many professional bodies agreed and seemed unconcerned about the proposals – indeed the BMA actively engaged with the process and initially went along with the proposed model whereby citizens would automatically have their data uploaded to a central database unless they actively opted out of the system. Given that there was very little publicity it was not surprising that very few did opt out. This fact was used by the government to justify care.data, but they neglected to mention they hadn't actually told people about it.

The government was eventually forced to undertake an 'information campaign' and every household was supposed to get a leaflet, for which the Royal Mail was paid over £1m.[39] Unfortunately the leaflets were often stuffed inside fliers for pizza shops and cruise brochures and ended up in the bin – so that many people were still none the wiser about care.data. Campaigners were angry that over £1m had been spent on a junk mail publicity campaign that had very little impact at a time when severe cuts were being made to frontline care elsewhere in the NHS.

The media became interested in the story and the public began to be concerned about their confidential information. They didn't trust the reassurances from governments who had in recent times shown themselves to be totally incompetent at keeping data confidential.[40] It became increasingly difficult for the HSCIC and government ministers to defend the opt out model and the fact that patients were so badly informed about the proposed medical data upload.

The final nail in the coffin came in January 2014 when *The Guardian* revealed that insurance companies, the pharmaceutical industry and other businesses could buy confidential patient medical data from the newly formed HSCIC to use for their own purposes. Mark Davies, HSCIC public assurance director, had to own up that there was a 'small risk' that harvested data could be identified down to individual patient level. He dismally failed to reassure patients by saying 'it depends on how people will use the data once they have it.'[41]

With pressure mounting from all quarters a decision was made in February 2014 to 'pause the process' of care.data and convene an expert advisory group to learn lessons and work out the next steps. In a sensible intervention Julia Hippisley-Cox, professor of general practice at Nottingham University, said 'there should be a clear audit trail that the patient can access and there needs to be a simple method for recording data sharing preferences and for these to be respected'.

Ministers and HSCIC leadership have yet to propose such a sensible approach to care.data – and suspicion about their intentions to make use of (and money from) patient data remains. With the Summary Care Record now being resurrected[42] there is potential for a great deal of confusion over the role of the SCR and care.data – but perhaps this is the aim of politicians. Create as much confusion as possible and then slip through contentious policies in the hope that few will notice.

Secret meetings

In September 2014 an alarming story emerged. News was leaked of secret meetings being held between the big five management consultants, multinational healthcare companies and Department of Health officials. Together they had formed the secretive Commissioning Support Industry Group (CSIG) who were looking to win £1bn worth of contracts to advise CCGs on purchasing patient care. The contracts involved would include drug purchasing, patient care reforms and outsourcing services to the private sector.[43]

UnitedHealth (UH), Simon Stevens' previous employer,[44] not only chaired the un-minuted meetings and provided the secretariat but had paid for senior health ministers to visit its care centres in the US on a five day 'fact finding mission'. Dr Chris Exeter, UH's UK lobbyist who had previously worked for a lobbying firm run by Andrew Lansley's wife, helped co-ordinate the meetings. The story was the final confirmation of NHS campaigners' fears – that far from GPs being at the heart of decision making, it would be management consultants and multinational healthcare corporations who held the NHS budgets and called the shots. The private sector would finally be in charge of advising about the purchase of NHS care from the private sector.

Lies

Type 'politicians lies NHS' into Google and pages of links come up. Successive governments have lied and lied again about the NHS and their intentions for it; they have had to. As Leys and Player point out in their book: 'If the public had been asked whether they wanted to see the NHS broken up – run for profit by a variety of multinational health companies, private equity funds and local businessmen, they would have overwhelmingly rejected it.'[45]

The lies have been necessary to conceal the true privatising agenda from the voting public, since as Portillo pointed out no one would have voted for it.* They have also been necessary to draw a veil over the vested interests looking to profit from the break-up of the NHS, and to cover up the damage done by the financial cuts (which they also lied about) and by Lansley's ill-conceived legislation. Egregious lies had to be

---

* A 2013 Yougov poll showed 84 per cent of the public would prefer to see the NHS run as a not-for-profit public service, while only 7 per cent favoured privatisation.

told about the NHS itself, and how it couldn't go on like this (see Chapter 2), lies necessary to justify their assault on the service.

We are now so inured to financial impropriety that we are apt to turn the page on yet another story about shady connections between politicians and the private sector. We are so accustomed to a diet of lies that we are hardly surprised when national institutions have to point out to our politicians that they are being economical with the facts. The UK Statistics Authority had to write to Jeremy Hunt pointing out that Tory claims of increased spending on the NHS were not true[46] but they went on lying anyway, with Cameron making further false claims about NHS spending.[47] Hunt (who had parliamentary form of course) was accused of repeated lying about various aspects of NHS performance.[48] As Leys and Player pointed out,[49] even the culture within the DoH itself changed from one of accountability and fidelity to one of misrepresentation and spin, which the authors attributed to the arrival of more private sector personnel in the department.

The biggest lie of all (and there are some serious contenders) was Cameron's pre-election promise that 'the NHS will be safe in my hands'. Far from being safe in Tory hands the NHS and its patients are now the victims of lies, profiteering, contracts for donors, jobs for the boys, the sale of confidential data and secret meetings run by a US multinational who is the ex-employer of the NHS CEO. No wonder they are so anxious that we don't know the facts about what is happening to the NHS.

Misleading the public
One of the most serious aspects of the lies and cover ups is

that the voting public does not have anywhere near the full facts to make up its mind about the political agenda for the NHS, which would allow them to call politicians account. The three major political parties have espoused the neoliberal ideology which demands marketisation of the NHS and as a result successive governments have ignored evidence and manipulated statistics to suggest that the NHS market is beneficial.

As Professor Calum Paton points out in his closely argued case against the marketisation of the NHS,[50] there has for example been no attempt to monitor the cost of the market reforms, allowing pro-marketeers to claim minor benefits while ignoring the expense incurred, which has been considerable. He calculates that the benefit-cost ratio of market reforms is likely to be very low at best and at worst a double negative i.e. high costs incurred in doing harm rather than in creating benefit. If politicians had been truthful about this we would long ago have recognised the English NHS market to be a failed experiment that has cost a great deal and delivered little. Based on the evidence, withheld from the public, it should have been abandoned years ago. Therein lies the real damage done by political lies, dishonesty and obfuscation.

12

Looking ahead

NHS reforms our worst mistake, Tories admit.[1]

The Times, October 2014

Where do we go from here?

We have set out in this book to chart the effects on the NHS of the Health and Social Care Act and of the cuts required by the Tory ten year plan to freeze NHS spending in real terms and reduce it as a share of GDP by 2020.[2] We have challenged the lies politicians have told us in order to push through their programme for marketising and privatising the NHS and to buttress their false claims that they have protected the NHS from funding cuts. From the preceding chapters it is clear that whoever wins the general election in May 2015 will face an NHS in serious crisis.

As this book has been drafted the scale of this crisis has grown and the pace of events has increased. We have massive and unsustainable pressure on secondary care while at the same time commissioners throughout England are drawing up plans to cut back hospital services, with ambitious hopes of diverting an ever-increasing number of patients away from hospitals and 'into the community'. Perhaps the most notable phenomenon has been the extension of so-called 'winter pressures' into all year round pressure on A&E and ambulance services, largely attributable to the near-collapse of social care after year-on-year reductions in local government spending.*

GPs and primary care services are also struggling, faced with a funding reduced in real terms and as a share of total NHS spending, while the tasks dumped onto GPs and primary care continue to increase with each new plan drawn up by Clinical Commissioning Groups (CCGs). The serious shortage of GPs to maintain services during the day and out of hours is matched by shortages of district nurses, other nursing staff and other health professionals.[3]

Short-sighted government and Department of Health decisions to run down training programmes for new health professionals are bearing bitter fruit. The problem is now compounded by the fact that the Health and Social Care Act carved up the responsibility for the education and training of health professionals into a myriad fragmented 'Local Education Training Boards',[4] just one example of the bureaucratic nightmare that Lansley's 'reforms' have unleashed on the NHS. Reports now suggest that up to 6,000 overseas nurses from other EU countries have been recruited in the year to date in attempts to plug the gaps created in the NHS workforce.[5]

The strains on acute services and primary care are matched by those afflicting mental health services, which despite increasing rhetoric from ministers have suffered years of disproportionately higher cuts than acute services, with loss of beds in hospitals alongside severe pressure on the replacement services in the community. Shortages

* As the book goes to press NHS Providers, representing 94 per cent of NHS hospitals, have dug their heels in and declared that enough is enough. They have refused to sign off their annual budget, claiming their members could no longer 'achieve the impossible' and that a fifth successive year of cuts would mean they could no longer guarantee the safe care of patients. http://www.theguardian.com/society/2015/jan/29/englands-biggest-hospitals-refuse-nhs-budget-patient-safety-fears.

of inpatient services* for child and adolescent mental health have hit the headlines,[6] while a less acknowledged bed shortage is also affecting the ability to deliver a full range of adult mental health services. Already the future of some specialist mental health care has been put at risk by incompetent commissioning from NHS England.[7]

Integrally linked into this mounting chaos has been the draconian 27 per cent cutback in local government funding over the five years to 2015,[8] which has necessarily impacted on social care, making it impossible in many areas to discharge patients from hospital, or to support vulnerable older people in their own homes. In many areas in England 'eligibility criteria' have been tightened to exclude almost all but the most serious and desperate cases from any support from social care. With council spending still falling and NHS budgets static in real terms, the illusion that services can somehow be 'integrated' by top slicing £3.5bn from NHS budgets to spend jointly with local authorities through the so-called 'Better Care Fund' has become even more far-fetched.

The *Health Service Journal* has warned that the ambitious targets set for the Better Care Fund are hopelessly unrealistic,[9] as the evidence accumulates to show that the obsessive focus on reducing attendances at A&E and emergency admissions is unlikely to yield significant results. So why do the plans for economies through reconfiguration of services focus so consistently on emergency services, which are relatively cheap to provide and consume such a relatively small share of the budget? When McKinsey produced their report for NHS London in 2009,[10] outlining savings proposals, their figures showed that spending on A&E (seeing 3.8 million patients)

---

* There have even been incidents of mentally unstable children locked up police cells overnight due to the shortage of adolescent beds. http:/www. theguardian.com/society/2014/aug/17/mentally-ill-children-police-cells.

was just £300m out of £11.3bn – just 2.6 per cent of London's health budget.

As we have seen in Chapter 10, when an A&E closes, it is the first step to the run-down and closure of the whole hospital, since so many other services are linked with A&E. The rationalisation of hospitals, to leave fewer and fewer emergency centres, also means that these remaining NHS hospitals will increasingly be dominated by emergency work, allowing the private sector to pick up yet more contracts to deliver the elective services which it finds most profitable.

PFI revisited

Another major problem in many areas is that dozens of trusts are facing a legacy of unaffordable contractual payments on costly PFI-funded hospitals. Deals which were unrealistic and barely affordable in the 2000s (when NHS spending grew year by year) are now proving to be major liabilities, consuming a large and growing proportion of the revenue of the parent trust. At the same time all acute hospitals face crippling financial challenges. These include annual cuts in the tariff of payments they receive for treatment, loss of income as CCGs attempt to reduce the numbers of patients referred to hospital, and competitive tenders which allow the private sector to take over significant amounts of elective care.

None of the main parties has offered any solution to the problems of hospitals burdened by Private Finance Initiative (PFI) repayments. The Tories enjoy pointing the finger of blame at Labour (at the same time as they are signing new PFI deals) while Ed Miliband continues to defend PFI and the disastrous decisions that were taken by Labour in the last decade.[11]

Debate continues among campaigners about how to tackle

the problem of PFI. Many campaigners instinctively reject any scheme that does not penalise the private consortia for having used their powerful position as 'the only game in town' to press-gang the NHS (which needed to build new hospitals) into signing overpriced contracts. But it's clear that the private sector lawyers have nailed down fairly watertight contracts, which are not easy to override without potentially costly legal challenges.[12]

It's also clear that even if it might save some money in the long term, most PFI contracts are too costly to be simply bought out, along the lines of a recent buyout for a small PFI in the north-east, where a local council was able to lend much of the money.[13] The discussion continues on a more substantial solution to the problem, but in the meantime action has to be taken to prevent PFI-driven financial pressures resulting in cuts in frontline services that harm patients. Public campaigns against PFI must start from the need to protect and maintain local services.

The process of educating the public, health workers, and even politicians about the inflated costs of many PFI schemes could start by demanding that all substantial PFI contracts be opened up to public scrutiny. This would happen alongside a process of renegotiation on the basis of fair value, which should in many cases result in reducing the outgoings year by year, and even the return of excessive payments to the NHS. Where cases can be proved, those responsible for misrepresenting facts and mis-selling PFI deals should face legal action.[14]

Deeper divisions between purchasers and providers
The Health and Social Care Act has deepened the division between commissioners (largely dominated by primary

care) and providers such as hospitals which are increasingly excluded from decision-making but obliged to cope with the consequences of decisions made elsewhere.

A snapshot survey of acute trusts and Clinical Commissioning Groups in London at the end of 2014 reveals the CCGs projecting an overall surplus of over £150m by April 2015 (despite some individual CCGs facing substantial deficits) while the acute trusts are projecting an overall deficit of more than £150m.[15] Some CCGs, confident of making a surplus, are nevertheless demanding penalty payments from local hospitals for exceeding contracted numbers of A&E patients and emergency admissions, while the CCGs themselves do nothing to reduce the pressures on these emergency services. This is a prime example of the so called beggar-my-neighbour behaviour which results in one section of the NHS trying to profit to the detriment of another and is a travesty of the traditional co-operation which used to characterise the NHS to the benefit of patients.

Simon Stevens' Five Year Forward View

In apparent contrast to the fragmentation and competition created by the Health and Social Care Act, Simon Stevens, the chief executive of NHS England, has published his 'vision' for the development of the English NHS over the next five years, which makes no reference to competition or to the private sector, but talks repeatedly about integration of services.[16] The Five Year Forward View has been welcomed by all three main political parties, each of which claims that it reflects their aspirations for the English NHS.

Others view the report as proposing a significant departure from the current model of the NHS, making radical changes that politicians dare not.[17] Critics have noted that new structures such as 'multi-speciality community providers' and 'primary and acute care systems' (PACs) are akin to accountable care organisations modelled on Kaiser Permanente, the US Health Maintenance Organisation (HMO). Some argue their appearance could prepare the way for an insurance based system for the NHS and allow private multinationals to run the NHS as US style HMOs and hospital chains.

Thus while *The Five Year Forward View* carefully skirts around any reference to competition or the free market established by the Health and Social Care Act, it contains avenues that could lead to further privatisation. It has indeed been labelled by some 'a wish list for privatisers',[18] 39 pages of sophisticated propaganda dressed up in bland language about 'integration' while containing hand grenades for the NHS. As described in Chapter 11, the contentious ideas are well concealed between layers of platitudes about the NHS and one has to dig deep to understand what is really being proposed.

Stevens concedes that the Tory plan to freeze NHS spending in real terms up to 2021 is unsustainable, but his answer is to call for a combination of £22bn of 'efficiency savings' over the five-year period – together with additional government funding of £8bn above inflation. There is little chance that either element of this ambitious equation will prove to be possible. There are serious doubts over the possibility of raising such substantial amounts of savings. All three main parties – even while welcoming the Stevens plan (which contains sufficient motherhood and apple pie to make criticism seem churlish) – have promised much smaller additional amounts towards the NHS budget than Stevens has requested. Stevens makes no mention of the many problems arising from the NHS market and its associated high costs, which should come as no surprise given his background of ten years as a senior executive at United Health, one of the biggest US healthcare multinationals.

Genuine integration is vital, even though Stevens has used the concept of 'integration' to dress up his new US-inspired models of care. One of our main criticisms of the Health and Social Care Act, competition and the market that has been created in health care since 2000 is that they fragment health services, restrict the proper integration of care and obstruct the planning of services to meet local needs. It's not integration that is the problem, but the potential role and influence of the private sector, and the fact that social care – funded through local government and not the NHS – has always been subject to means-tested charges (and in recent years almost entirely delivered by private sector contractors) and not, as the NHS, provided free at point of use and funded from general taxation.

This is why any progressive integration of health and social care must be led by the NHS, publicly owned and financed, and not handed over to local government on its present rules. There must also be a campaign for the abolition of means-tested charges and for proper funding of social care, as well as improved wages and conditions for care staff, many of whom are on zero hours contracts and near the minimum wage. It's time to bring social care services back into public ownership and control.

Throughout *The Five Year Forward View* document Stevens clearly places heavy reliance on an expanded role for health promotion and prevention of ill-health to reduce the demand on frontline services that would in turn result in savings. While every sensible person is in favour of improving public health, avoiding the excessive use of hospitals and healthcare interventions, and minimising dependence on drugs, any strategy based on health promotion is necessarily going to take a long time before it delivers tangible results, and will make little if any significant short-term difference to the needs of older vulnerable patients for hospital and other health care. Indeed life expectancy has fallen slightly in some parts of England since 2011, the first time this has happened in many years.[19] Cuts to social services and pressures on the NHS have been blamed.

How much of the NHS is there left to fight for?

On 1 October 2014, Cambridgeshire and Peterborough Clinical Commissioning Groups announced that the biggest contracting exercise to date had concluded by awarding an £800m, five-year contract for Older Peoples Services not, as feared, to Virgin or Care UK, both on the final shortlist, but to the NHS bid, headed by Cambridge University Hospitals NHS Foundation Trust.[20]

It was a timely reminder that despite the irresponsible actions of some CCGs, tendering exercises do not have to result in privatisation. However they DO inevitably waste huge amounts of money and management time, disrupt cooperative and collaborative working relationships with local providers, and create more complex and less stable systems.

Elsewhere tendering exercises have resulted in worse outcomes. As discussed in Chapter 8, companies and private-led consortia have been picking up contracts that seriously destabilise local provision of core NHS services. Private sector inroads are disproportionately disruptive, even if their scale is frequently exaggerated. The damage to the NHS as a single, comprehensive service, which should be planned around local health needs rather than subject to a maelstrom of competitive markets, goes much further than the amount of money involved.*

In fact the private sector has never shown any ambition to take over the whole of the NHS, in the way private capital once coveted British Telecom, British Gas, and other utilities. The reason for this is simple: as discussed in Chapters 8 and 9, the private sector is profit-hungry but largely risk-averse. Most of the NHS is high risk, and not profitable in its current form. It can only be made attractive to the private sector by paying over the odds for services which the NHS currently provides at lower cost – and thus inflating costs – or by excluding risk, for example by refusing to cover more complex and costly cases.

Private companies want only the sectors of the NHS which they (sometimes wrongly) believe offer the prospects of delivering simple, uncomplicated services for guaranteed profits. But their narrow focus of interest means that their perhaps surprisingly small total share of the cake has become far more significant than it might appear. A Department of Health spokesman said in September 2014: 'Use of the private sector in the NHS represents only 6 per cent of the total NHS budget [£6.3bn] – an increase of just 1 per cent since May 2010.'[21] Much of the budget for patient care, however, consists of services that the private sector does not, and does not wish to, provide. Their main interest, apart from social care, is concentrated in elective care, community health services

* The privatisation of hospital cleaning and other support services back in the 1980s has become almost universally recognised as a disastrous race to the bottom on quality of services. It wasn't until Tony Blair's government took office that serious attempts were made to hand NHS clinical services to the private sector.

and mental health - the main growth areas up to now. So the £6.3bn needs to be seen not as a share of the *total* spend, but as a proportion of the *relevant* spending in the NHS. (For this and other reasons private providers cause disproportionate damage. What is more, the Health and Social Care Act has been in place for only two years, so the story is just beginning).

So more precisely, the £6.3bn in private clinical contracts are focused on £48bn of the NHS budget involving the areas of interest to the private sector (primary care, mental health, community and elective services). That means 13.2 per cent of this sector of the NHS is now contracted out to profit-seeking private companies.

But let's not forget that the remaining, crucial 86.8 per cent is still (for the time being) in the public sector – along with virtually all of the other clinical services, and 100 per cent of the costly, complex and emergency caseload. This is no argument for complacency: figures show that up to a third of new contracts have been going to the private sector and another substantial share to the voluntary sector, leaving just 55 per cent of new contracts retained within the NHS.[22]

As discussed in Chapter 9, there have been some local-level inroads into primary care and contracts for general practice (one profit-seeking company with 20-plus practices in Merseyside, for example) and in particular out of hours contracts. Overall the contract value of corporate provision of primary care remains small in comparison with the total spend, and the contracts have often been short-lived, struggling to recruit and retain appropriately skilled staff on terms and conditions less favourable than mainstream primary care.

The Institute of Fiscal Studies concluded from its 2013 analysis of figures up to 2012: 'Despite large growth in the role of private providers in the delivery of some procedures, the vast majority of care is still provided by NHS hospitals.'[23] The impact of tendering is not evenly spread because not every area has contracted this work to private providers. In some areas the private sector has made little headway, in others it has a disproportionate share of uncomplicated elective care.

As noted in Chapter 5, the impact on those NHS and foundation trust hospitals which are affected is magnified by the fact that the private sector takes only the least complex elective services, leaving the NHS with all the more costly complex patients as well as the emergencies. This results in a reduced overall caseload, and thus less income with which to maintain services. It also poaches staff trained by the NHS at public expense and, by taking routine cases, the private sector creates problems for teaching hospitals in training a new generation of doctors and specialist nurses – since the private sector provides no training, and runs an atypical case mix and environment unsuitable for training.

More damage has also been done in community services, where the private sector has won contracts mostly on the basis of loss leaders, and has so far largely failed to deliver any of the hoped-for profits. As they try to extract profits from what were previously often under-funded and neglected services, the private sector scales down the workforce, dilutes the skill mix, and often runs into serious recruitment and retention problems. This is one reason why Serco, previously one of the market leaders, have recently pulled out of contracting, having withdrawn early from some existing contracts, admitting to substantial losses. Other leading companies are known to have serious problems.[24]

But as Chapter 9 recounts, musculoskeletal (MSK) and other contracts are still being tendered by some CCGs. Among the most irresponsible is NHS Kernow, which is putting elective services out to tender that are worth a quarter of the Royal Cornwall Hospital Trust's budget – despite the fact that this could seriously destabilise the only acute hospital provider in the giant peninsula county.[25] So the overall share of these service budgets going private could still be set to increase significantly, especially if the Tories win the next election. The trend since 2010, as the NHS Support Federation has shown, has been towards private sector providers.

But let's not forget that even in elective and community services (which are most affected by privatisation) and mental health, where 14 per cent or more of spending goes to private providers, the vast majority of services – including all of the crucial emergency services and care for chronic and complex cases – are still in the hands of providers rooted in the NHS, and run not for profit. There is plenty of the NHS left to fight for and much to try to recapture.

The Cambridgeshire decision shows that privatisation is NOT a necessary and inevitable conclusion of even the skewed tendering process imposed by the Health and Social Care Act. The level of public awareness, and the resultant local outcry at privatisation, a factor that clearly influenced the Cambridgeshire decision, are growing. The summer of 2014 saw 300-strong meetings in Stoke on Trent to challenge the possible privatisation of the pathways for cancer and end of life care in Staffordshire.[26]

A reversal of the Act, along the lines of the NHS Reinstatement Bill[27] would therefore open the door to reclaiming the remainder of the services as contracts come to an end, or private companies themselves follow Serco and pull out for lack of adequate profits.

Some generic principles for the NHS

Forests have been felled in the pursuit of writing about better ways to run the NHS and we do not intend to add to them with this book, but a number of suggestions have already been put forward which are brought together here for convenience:

- The Secretary of State should take back responsibility for the NHS.
- There is no place for a competitive market in delivering health care. The purchaser provider split has been an expensive and failed experiment and should be scrapped.
- Patient choice should be choice that is relevant to patients and not politically expedient. Individual patient choice has consequences which have to be weighed against civic responsibility.
- Patient voice is important for the health of the NHS and should be restored via structures commanding the same degree of influence as Community Health Councils once did.
- The NHS must be adequately funded by international comparators. Significant amounts of money can be saved by ending the competitive market and dealing with the loss of money to PFI projects. Opinion polls show that the public is willing to fund a publicly provided NHS via a hypothecated tax[28] (i.e. specific taxation producing revenue for particular expenditure.): but the bulk of the cost should flow from collecting the £120bn of unpaid tax each year[29] and other progressive taxation.
- There should be a culture of learning from errors rather than naming and shaming.
- There needs to be proper investment in NHS staff and their training.

- The main job of managers should be to facilitate clinical activity and not to chase political targets.

Healthy competition is possible

A final broad brush suggestion for getting better results from the NHS is an experiment conducted many years ago by a Dutch teaching hospital in Maastricht in an attempt to improve referrals to the hospital. They wrote new guidelines for referring patients for imaging and pathology, and circulated them to the local GPs, who were at the same time given an identifying number. The hospital then fed back anonymised data to the GPs which showed how well they had done in adhering to the guidelines. They could only identify their own number in the data, which allowed then to see how well they had done in relation to others, but to remain anonymous to others.

The interesting result was that everyone's referral behaviour improved. There was no financial incentive, no naming and shaming, only professional pride to motivate the doctors to improve their performance, and they did. Once they knew via the feedback how they were doing in comparison with their peers they were motivated to improve, although no one else knew how well or badly they had done.

Professionals by and large are not interested in competing on a financial basis but are easily motivated by professional pride. Nobody sets out in the morning to do a bad day's work but the NHS has never exploited the natural pride that health professionals have in doing a good job. This is something that has been largely overlooked by management consultants, politicians and others who speak endlessly of 'incentivising' professionals, usually with non-clinical incentives such as targets-with-menaces. We would like to suggest that the appropriate bodies look at this as a matter of urgency, as it offers a benign way of encouraging healthy competition that would benefit both staff and patients and save money at the same time.*

The political outlook

As the book goes to press we are weeks away from the 2015 general election. The outcome is less than clear but whatever the result the next government will inherit an NHS in genuine crisis. As we hope we have shown in the book, there was no need for this, as the NHS was doing very well until the advent of the coalition government, and its current problems can largely be traced to misjudged political interference and inadequate funding.

Many would like to vote for a party that will commit to an NHS that is not artificially divided into buyers and sellers of care, and where collaboration replaces competition, but that is still not a real possibility. All three major parties are still committed to the purchaser-provider split and with that come greater or lesser degrees of competition and outsourcing, depending on the particular party.

Labour, of course, have said they will reverse much of the legislation and promote the NHS to the status of 'preferred provider' which would be a step in the right direction. But one of the authors was recently told by a senior Labour official that it was necessary to maintain the purchaser-provider split because competition was 'good for the NHS'. It was alarming to hear that such a belief is still held by highly placed people in the Labour party, but old attitudes are deeply entrenched.

* One of the authors was part of an application for a grant to carry out the same experiment at a London teaching hospital, which was turned down. How different things might have been if that lesson had been taken on board for the English NHS.

Labour unfortunately built the bridge across which the Tories have stormed the NHS and there are still too many at the heart of the party who don't think they did anything wrong when they destabilised the service by vigorously promoting its marketisation.

The Greens have adopted a very progressive health policy[30] which includes calling for the scrapping of the Health and Social Care Act, and opposing the whole of the US-EU Transatlantic Trade and Investment Partnership treaty.

The National Health Action Party, much more recently arrived on the scene, have drawn up an ambitious policy framework,[31] starting from the need to combat austerity and neoliberalism, and putting the fight for repeal of the Health and Social Care Act and scrapping the competitive market in the NHS in this context. The National Health Action Party supports the Pollock-Roderick NHS Reinstatement Bill,[32] calls for significant increases in NHS funding, and is consistently opposed to PFI and all forms of privatisation.

With the spark of political resistance and alternative policies on offer from these and other progressive critics of Labour's official line, the chances of campaigners fighting back long after the general election are greatly increased. It's only by understanding what is happening and fighting tooth and nail against each attack as it comes that our NHS can be defended, reinstated and developed to fulfil its role as our most popular and universal public service, free to all at point of need, offering a full range of treatment, run for patients, not for profit, and funded from taxation.

NHS for sale

As this chapter is completed the latest casualty of the push to privatisation is Hinchingbrooke Hospital, whose takeover by the private firm Circle is described in Chapter 1. Circle, who had promised unrealistic levels of savings in order to win the contract, have announced that they are pulling out after only three years of their ten-year term. They have said their continuing involvement was 'unsustainable', blaming funding cuts, social care shortages and a surge in demand for A&E services – conditions which the NHS faces every day and is expected to deal with, not having the private sector's option of walking away. As angry tweeters remarked – when the going gets tough, the private sector gets going. It was no coincidence that on the day Circle announced their decision they received a damning report from the Care Quality Commission, of which they had been previously notified. It revealed a catalogue of serious failings and resulted in Hinchingbrooke being the first hospital ever found to be 'inadequate' in how it cares for patients. Circle blamed anybody and everybody and their shares fell by 25 per cent. An unseemly political row broke out over who had awarded the contract in the first place. The NHS was as usual left to sort out the mess.[33]

Supporters of Circle's role at Hinchingbrooke weren't slow to comment on the turn of events. Jeremy Hunt tweeted 'This [government] makes no apology for seeking solutions for failing hospitals. We won't be deterred from tackling poor care and driving up standards.'[34] Not even by the biggest private sector flop to date it seems. The *Daily Mail* predictably sprang to Circle's defence. It had been a staunch champion of the takeover, claiming that Circle had turned the hospital from a 'basket case' to best in country for patient care.[35] They explained away its failure to live up to their headlines by suggesting that the hospital was the victim of a 'stitch up' by opponents of private enterprise in the NHS and scooped the fact that one of the 35-strong Care Quality Commission team was possibly a member of the campaign group Keep Our NHS Public, a sure sign of skulduggery.[36]

Critics of NHS privatisation were quick to claim that Circle's failure sounded the death knell for the private sector in the NHS, but although it is too early to be sure the lesson is almost certainly a different one. Private companies will want even less to do with the risky and unprofitable end of the NHS, including District General Hospitals, and will gravitate ever more to the profitable activity, including administrative and policy support for the unnecessary market, leaving the complex expensive work[37] for the NHS to pick up.*

The story of Hinchingbrooke, outsourced to and then badly failed by the private sector, seems a suitable place to rest our case. We hope that this book, with its evidence against competition, the NHS market and all the trappings that go with it, will finally kill the NHS market zombie. The NHS will always need to evolve and improve, but the direction of travel that all three major parties have adopted for it over the last twenty years has been an expensive failure in terms of actual money wasted and in terms of high opportunity costs. The billions wasted on marketising the NHS could and should have been spent on patient care.**

The deleterious effects of the policies pushed through to enforce a market extend far beyond the contracts awarded to the private sector and the money diverted to them. They

---

* It would be an irony if the clinical market – meant to give patients choice – were to be increasingly abandoned by the private sector in order to concentrate on running the self-same market in which they are by and large no longer interested.
** Those who want a full analysis of the truly shocking amount of money wasted on the NHS market in England are referred to Calum Paton's excellent paper for CHPI 'At what cost? Paying the price for the market in the English NHS' from http://chpi.org.uk/.

have a profound effect on the core of the NHS (which will always be required to deliver the services of no interest to the private sector), undermining services, destabilising NHS trusts as elective care is lost to the private sector and diverting scarce clinical time and resources away from patient care into dealing with the demands of compulsory competitive tendering and unbridled competition. The result is money squandered, opportunities lost and harm to the system which we all rely on.

The NHS needs stability and adequate funding, which would allow it to address the real problems it faces – tackling health inequalities, improving clinical standards, training enough staff, determining the appropriate distribution of care between hospitals and the community. The NHS market is a costly distraction for which there is no evidence, an ideological luxury which we cannot afford, above all in a time of 'austerity'. It's time to end the failed market experiment and return to an NHS which is publicly funded, publicly provided and publicly accountable.

For the last word we return to Noam Chomsky, who neatly identified how politicians and big business collude to put popular public services like the NHS 'up for sale'

That's the standard technique of privatisation: defund, make sure things don't work, people get angry, you hand it over to private capital.[38]

It's our job to make sure they don't get away with it.

The Health Lobbying Industry

TAMASIN CAVE

In the run up to the general election of 2010, David Cameron made a pitch to the electorate that spoke directly to voter frustration with our broken political system. Lobbying, he said, specifically 'secret corporate lobbying … goes to the heart of why people are so fed up with politics.'[1] He pointed to public 'fears and suspicions' about how our political system works, with 'money buying power, power fishing for money and a cosy club at the top making decisions in their own interest'. 'We all know how it works,' he confidently assumed.

When it comes to the sell-off of the NHS, our fears and suspicions are well-founded. The views of the public towards the NHS have been sidelined as something to be managed by government rather than actively considered. Public opinion has largely been replaced in policy debates by corporate wish lists.

How the private healthcare lobby won the ear of government, however, goes well beyond Cameron's gentle vision of lobbying: 'the lunches, the hospitality, the quiet word in your ear'. The lobbying assault on the NHS by private healthcare interests has been a well-resourced effort over successive governments, involving multiple, overlapping strategies. It has included the financing of political parties, think tanks and very many lobby groups; the manipulation of public debate through the press; the 'revolving door' and the capture of whole government institutions by pro-market players; as well as the old-fashioned, behind-closed-doors schmoozing as described by Cameron.

Let us initially concentrate on the lobbying efforts of just one corporation by way of an illustration (or at least the lobbying that is known to us). UnitedHealth Group is a giant in American healthcare. As well as being one of the largest private health insurers in the US, it has a fast growing business in technology-driven health services. It is involved in the commissioning (or buying) of health services, in outsourcing, and in the promotion of 'wellbeing' services to consumers, including through wearable technology.[2] Revenue for the group in 2013 hit $122bn.[3]

The company is not without its critics in the US where it has faced accusations of overcharging and malpractice.[4] Every year it spends millions of dollars on political donations and Washington lobbyists.[5] Its ambitions, though, extend across the pond and, in the past decade, the firm has secured multiple NHS contracts. It is now in the running for what is thought to be the biggest outsourcing deal in NHS history, the £1.2bn contract to run cancer and end-of-life services across Staffordshire.[6]

UnitedHealth is, in its own words, 'committed to creating a strategic partnership with the NHS at various levels'.[7] Time and money have been invested in building relationships with UK decision-makers to achieve this aim. For instance, it has courted senior health officials, flying them on all-expenses-paid trips to its US headquarters and facilities. The purpose of a five-day junket in 2014 was for British officials to understand how the 'innovations and experience' of this US insurance giant might help inform the development of the NHS.[8]

UnitedHealth has also led the way in securing itself a seat inside the NHS. In mid 2014, it was discovered that the US corporation chairs a discreet forum of private companies that has been granted regular access to senior NHS officials and briefings on policies in which they have a commercial interest. Members of the group, which also includes KPMG, PwC, Capita and McKinsey, are competing for nearly £1bn of NHS contracts advising GP groups on how to spend their two-thirds share of the NHS budget. The group is co-ordinated by UnitedHealth's chief lobbyist, Chris Exeter.[9]

This moves us on to another aspect of UnitedHealth's lobbying: the hiring of well-connected insiders. Exeter is a former health official who, for a period around 2011, worked for the lobbying firm run by the wife of NHS reformer-in-chief, ex-health secretary Andrew Lansley.[10] Exeter's predecessor at the firm, Tony Sampson, was a Number 10 health policy advisor and private secretary to another pro-market health secretary, now PwC health advisor, Alan Milburn.[11]

For the past five years, UnitedHealth has also bought in extra lobbying firepower in the form of lobbying agency Hanover Communications, which is similarly well-connected in health policy circles.[12] Not only has the agency recently been employed by NHS England,[13] Hanover's health practice is also headed up by Andrew Harrison, an ex-health official and a former close colleague of Simon Stevens, the current chief executive of the NHS.[14] Then, of course, there is Stevens. Before returning to lead the NHS in 2014, he had spent nearly a decade working in the US for UnitedHealth.

There are, in addition to this, the very many lobbying groups of which UnitedHealth is a paid up member. These lobbyists have done a lot of the leg work to ensure the recent controversial changes to the NHS stay on track. The industry lobby group, the NHS Partners Network, for example, successfully lobbied for an official inquiry that publicly reprimanded 'maverick' local commissioners who were intent on keeping the health service public (or who were 'unreasonably restricting patients' choice' in the eyes of private health companies).[15] The Network, on behalf of its members, also secured an inside track when it came to the government's public consultation on its market reforms. It had private channels through which it could lobby both those that were supposed to be listening to public concerns and Number 10.[16] The Network has also been a vocal defender of the for-profit sector in the press. On one occasion it orchestrated, with the free-market think tank Reform, the placing of a sequence of articles in *The Telegraph* that warned the government not to let up on NHS privatisation.[17]

UnitedHealth is also a corporate partner and donor to Reform, which has pushed hard to win Parliamentarians and the public round to the government's health agenda.[18] The think tank has substantial political clout: Reform's deputy director, Nick Seddon, for example, moved on to become the Prime Minister's health advisor. Its spokespeople are also regular champions of more competition in the NHS in the pages of our newspapers. In order to reach an even broader audience with its message, Reform also provided support for a 'front group' called Doctors for Reform. Its GP spokesperson sought to win round public opinion on, for instance, the popular BBC Radio 2 lunchtime Jeremy Vine show. The commercial interests behind the group, however, were never revealed to Vine's five mIllion listeners.[19]

Another organisation that UnitedHealth sponsors is the Cambridge Health Network. This is an elite club for NHS leaders to meet and informally discuss policies with the for-profit health sector. Its regular talks, social events and private dinners provide, it says, 'a place where business connections and relationships are forged'.[20] Simon Stevens delivered both the inaugural speech at the network's first event in 2004, and on the occasion of its tenth anniversary.[21] Access to this 'confidential, closed forum', however, is granted only to those who pass the strict vetting procedure of the network's founders.

One of the co-founders, Penny Dash,[22] is a partner at international management consultancy firm, McKinsey, which is also one of the club's sponsors. The network has a commercial partner too, lobbying firm ZPB Partners, run by the wife of Simon Steven's colleague, NHS England director and McKinsey alumnus, Tim Kelsey.[22] Indeed, the Cambridge Health Network is seen by some as 'essentially a McKinsey front', one that provides valuable opportunities for private health companies and financial institutions to access and influence health officials.[23] McKinsey itself, though, is in no such need. The US firm has long been embedded in our health system and for decades has played a central role in the reform of the NHS.

During the latest shakeup, McKinsey could be found advising officials on the reforms at every level of the system: inside the Department of Health, NHS England and the regulator, Monitor, as well as being paid many millions by the newly-formed local commissioning groups and commissioning support units around the country. From April 2013-14, for example, McKinsey earned over £2.5m advising Monitor and £2.7m from NHS England, which included in excess of £1m for advice on health services in just one corner of London.[24]

McKinsey alumni today also find themselves in positions of significant influence: there are two at the helm of Monitor; one among only eight executive directors of NHS England; the chair of the Health and Social Care Information Centre (public custodians of our health data), as well as hospital chiefs and other key posts. The firm also hosts Department of Health meetings in their London offices, flies NHS officials on all expenses paid trips abroad, takes public servants and their families to West End shows, and entertains them at parties in exclusive venues like the National Gallery.[25]

McKinsey, however, devotes more of its energy to – and earns most of its revenue from – advising corporations: health insurers, private hospital groups, pharmaceutical companies, tech interests and investors. As the Coalition was embarking on its changes to the NHS, McKinsey was already gathering its thinking on the implications of the reforms and had 'started to share this with clients', it wrote.[26] The firm also appears to be acting as a bridge between the public and private sectors. Internal emails from the Department of Health show McKinsey connecting the capital's health officials with one of Germany's largest private hospital chains, Helios, to discuss 'potential opportunities' to take over public hospitals in London. McKinsey also advised them how to minimise public resistance to the privatisation of hospitals: start 'from a mindset [of] one at a time,' it warned.[27]

McKinsey is famously tight-lipped about its private sector clients. Who they work for and what they do for them is confidential. It is not the only firm that occupies this powerful position, though, as advisers to both government and corporations, where the potential for conflicts of interest exists. The Big Four accountancy giants are in the business too.

Take KPMG. Its public sector work includes earning £3.5m in the seven months to March 2014 from the NHS bodies set up to provide commissioning services to GP groups.[28] It is receiving, for instance, just shy of £200,000 a month from the Greater East Midlands commissioning support unit for consultancy and other services.[29] KPMG is also part of a consortium led by UnitedHealth that is in the running for an estimated £1bn of contracts in the same NHS market, providing these same commissioning support services.[30]

At the same time, KPMG is engaged with the private healthcare sector. Addressing a conference of healthcare companies and investors in New York in 2010, Mark Britnell, head of KPMG's UK health division, spoke of the private sector opportunities presented by the UK's health reforms: 'The NHS will be shown no mercy and the best time to take advantage of this will be in the next couple of years,' he advised the attending companies. These included BUPA, private hospital firms, HCA and Netcare, and UnitedHealth.[31] Britnell was speaking a year into his job at KPMG, which he joined from the Department of Health where he was director general in charge of commissioning.

Another of the Big Four, PwC, has similarly picked up many millions of pounds in consultancy work from across the public system. At the same time, PwC is looking to increase its position in what it sees as the UK's growing, commercial market in healthcare. Tasked with this job is its Health Industry Oversight Board. This industry panel is chaired by former health secretary, Alan Milburn, just one of a long list of former ministers from across the political parties to now employ their expertise in the private sector.[32]

* * *

The 'cosy club at the top' that Cameron referred to should now be starting to come into view. The picture that emerges is of a largely corporate-funded closed network, peopled by commercial players, senior officials at the top of the NHS and their former colleagues, lobbyists, think tanks and social networks, all operating with minimal public scrutiny.

This is by design. As one lobbyist notes: 'The influence of lobbyists increases when ... it goes largely unnoticed by the public.'[33] Officials and politicians have more room to negotiate when their actions are not being scrutinised by the press. Also deliberate are efforts by lobbyists to occupy a public official's environment, with invitations of corporate hospitality, social events, trips to facilities and discussions of ideas. The goal, over time, is that both parties – public and private – come to share the same set of values: the values of the market.

Above is just an outline of some of the access and influence enjoyed by just a few of the players in the UK's healthcare market. Imagine them now being joined by lobbyists from the pharmaceutical industry. Swiss drug giant Novartis, for example, employs a dozen lobbying firms in the UK on top of its in-house team, including one established by Andrew Lansley's former right-hand man, Bill Morgan.[34] Then there are the countless patient groups funded by the drug companies that are seen by the industry as the 'foot soldiers' in its lobbying battles with government.[35] The influential lobby group, the Association of the British Pharmaceutical Industry, even shares a building with NHS England, stewards of the £110bn NHS budget.

Add to these the construction companies and banks lobbying for more PFI deals; the private hospital companies seeking to expand their reach in the UK; the medical technology firms, the IT and telecoms giants, the private equity companies and investors. All of them have a commercial interest in the government's sweeping changes to the NHS. They also all have lobbyists with political connections; are part of lobbying groups that petition government; are invited in to advise government; employ press officers and fund think tanks to shape public debate.

There is no way for the public to know the scale of the various lobbies, who is involved, or how much money has been spent pushing for the dismantling of our public health service. Unlike the US and Canada, the UK has no disclosure rules that require lobbyists to operate in the open. In the UK we only ever get a glimpse of what they are up to. But, if we did know, if discussions between private health interests and government were in plain view, we might choose to join in. We might probe and challenge their assertions. We might agree with their solutions, or we might not. Our priorities might be the same or different from theirs. But crucially, we could begin to have the public debate we deserve as taxpayers on where the NHS is heading. Rest assured, discussions are being had, we are just not party to them.

A round-up of NHS vital statistics under the coalition

PAUL EVANS, NHS Support Federation

With thanks to Sylvia Davidson and Doug King Spooner

Many of the following fact and figures have already been covered elsewhere in the book and are gathered together and summarised here for ease of reference. They tell a powerful and depressing story and demonstrate that the policies that governments adopt can seriously undermine the NHS, sometimes making it seem as though the body itself is broken. The challenge is to recognise this and to transfer to policies that make the most of NHS strengths and further exploit its potential to provide care for us all.

1. What's the evidence that the NHS is being privatised?

The government does not hold central data on who has been awarded contracts to provide care to NHS patients. They say this because it is all organised locally. So to find out who is winning NHS contracts and pinpoint where public money is going takes considerable research.

Tracking NHS contracts

The NHS Support Federation has been monitoring the official website where tenders are advertised to find out which clinical services are being organised through the market. We followed this up with Freedom of information request to the clinical commissioning groups.[1]

This is a summary of our most recent investigation (October 2014) into the trends in NHS contract activity around clinical services. It covers the 18-month period since the Health and Social Care Act came into effect. By recording details from live contract adverts we have been able to track which services are open to private providers, which providers are winning contracts and how much money is involved.

Summary – NHS Clinical Contract Data
April 2013 to October 2014

1. Contracts to run or manage clinically related NHS services have been advertised in 865 notices in the first 18 months since the HSC Act came in to effect in April 2013. These have a combined value of £18.3bn over their lifetime.
2. £5bn worth of contracts have been awarded through the market since April 2013.
3. 67 per cent of these clinical awards have been won by non-NHS providers – totalling £2.4bn in value. A further £760m was shared in ten joint contracts.
4. £13bn remain in the pipeline. This is very likely an under estimate as around a third of tender adverts do not publicly reveal their contract value. However we estimate that non-NHS bodies stand to gain £6.6bn from the contracts still in the pipeline, if they continue to win contracts at the current rate (50 per cent of the total value tendered).
5. The number of NHS contracts being awarded through the market is rising significantly. In the first six months since the HSC Act came into effect (April-September 2013) over £400m of NHS contracts were awarded. A year later the number of awards (72) in the same six-month period (April-September 2014) has doubled and their value is over seven times higher, at £3bn.

6. A huge range of services are involved in these contracts. Overall we have counted over 80 categories of NHS service covering every aspect of the patient journey including diagnosis, treatment and ongoing health care across every possible setting. In 2012 there were just 40 types of treatment covered by contract notices.

7. The value of clinical notices placed by CCGs since April 2013 is £8bn – 604 contracts (many containing multiple commissioners). So far non-NHS providers have won 56 per cent of clinical awards from CCGs.

8. The most frequently advertised types of service (including Any Qualified Provider scheme) in terms of contract notices are Diagnostics (133), Mental Health (64), GP Services/out-of-hours/111 (59), Pharmacy (51) and Community Care (39).

9. In terms of value of contract notices plus awards, Community Care services were of the greatest value at just over £1.9bn, followed by Diagnostics at £1.2bn, then Elective Surgery at just over £1bn, MSK on £785m, patient transport/ambulance £583m and pharmacy £558m.

10. There has been a trend towards the use of the Prime Provider contract model, which involves the appointment of a single provider, which will then appoint subcontractors to carry out some of the work. This has been most noticeable in the area of MSK services where, from April 2013 to the end of September 2014, £709m worth of work has been awarded via prime provider contracts.

11. The largest contract for work within the NHS advertised since April 2013 is the *Framework for Commissioning Support Services* with a value of £3-5bn over a four-year period.

Primary Care

For several years GP surgeries and health centres have been gradually acquired by profit driven companies, such as Virgin Care, The Practice, and Care UK. Many patients may not be aware that their GP service is run by a private company.[2]

Together the top five private companies in the area of GP surgeries own 170 GP surgeries, with the leading company, SSP Health based in the north-west of England owning 42 surgeries, closely followed by The Practice PLC with 39 surgeries. Other top owners are Virgin Health, Malling Health and IntraHealth. With the exception of Virgin Health, all these companies have increased their ownership of GP surgeries from 2010 to 2014, and in the case of SSP Health, Malling Health and The Practice PLC, the number owned has more than doubled.

Emergency and out-of-hours care

Today, if you call 999 it could be a private ambulance crew that comes to treat you. For several years the NHS has been outsourcing the transport of patients but contracts are now being won by private companies to provide blue light services. Spending on private firms to provide 999 ambulances has doubled in the last three years from £24m to £56m.[3]

GP out of hours contracts are a priority for commissioners to put out to tender. Serco currently organises GP out of hours care services in Cornwall, but will quit the contract following criticism of quality of care.[4] Care UK (Harmoni) claims to cover 8 million NHS patients as part of its GP out of hours services. It also runs GP-led health centres, referral management centres, 111 telephone services, offender healthcare, and urgent care for the NHS.[5]

Community health services

Contracts to provide community healthcare typically cover a wide range of services including complex health needs of children and older people. Some CCGs have bundled these services into a single giant tender. Examples include, Virgin Care's £130m contract to run children's services, and services for people with learning difficulties and adolescents with mental health problems in Devon from March 2013 for three years and its £450m contract to run a range of community services in Surrey. More recently in July 2014, North Somerset CCG published a contract notice seeking bidders to provide an integrated community care service. The five year contract is valued at a maximum of £120m.[6]

Surgery

Private hospitals share of NHS-funded patients grew rapidly between 2006-7 and 2010-11 after the introduction of patient choice and as part of the ISTC programme. By 2010-11 private companies performed 17 per cent of hip replacements (11,500 operations), 17 per cent of hernia repairs (9,000) and 6 per cent of gall bladder removals (3,000) annually in England. By 2010-11 private providers also handled 8 per cent of patients' first attendances in relation to orthopaedics or trauma, such as a broken limb; 4.8 per cent of gastroenterological problems; and 2.3 per cent of attendances for sight problems. The latest figures from the HSCIC (2014) show that 12 per cent of all NHS cataract operations are now performed by private providers.

In 2012-13, 45,379 cataract operations were carried out by non-NHS providers, or 12.6 per cent of cataract procedures conducted overall. This is up from 10.6 per cent carried out by non-NHS providers in 2012-13.[7]

Non-NHS providers conducted 4 per cent of procedures

overall in 2013-14 or 437,919 up from 3.7 per cent in 2012-13 (388,211).[8]

There are now 195 independent hospitals and treatment centres in England where patients can be treated at NHS prices under the Choose and Book system. The total cost of contracting out runs into billions of pounds but the government has not published precise figures.[9]

Cancer care

In July 2014, four clinical commissioning groups in Stafford-shire tendered for a £687m, 10-year contract to provide cancer care, the first such contract in this area opened up to private companies.[10] The four CCGs involved are also seeking bidders for a separate £340m ten year contract to provide end-of-life care.[11] Together the contracts are worth £1.04bn. It has been reported that Virgin, Care UK, Ramsay Health and other private companies have all expressed interest in the contract. The *Health Service Journal* revealed that Lockheed Martin, which makes fighters for the RAF and Merlin helicopters for the Royal Navy, attended a meeting hosted by NHS England for firms interested in the contract.[12]

Commissioning Support Services

Locally each new GP-led CCG will be assisted by a Commissioning Support Unit (CSU). Each CSU covers a number of CCGs and they are already forging links with the private sector. The NHS Supply Chain has been run by the German logistics company DHL and NHS Shared Business Services (SBS), handling a wide range of back office functions, is 50 per cent owned by French IT company Sopra Steria. Private players involved in commissioning of services, include NHS SBS and the private company HealthTrust Europe, owned by the US hospital giant HCA. The *Financial Times* reported in November 2013 that private equity companies have been approached about the possibility of taking over or merging with 19 commissioning support units (CSUs).[13] In February 2014, NHS England issued a contract notice for £5bn seeking companies to compete for work advising CSUs; in early 2015 the winners are due to be announced, but companies such as Serco, Optum (part of UnitedHealth) and Assura are reported to have submitted expressions of interest.[14]

Hospital management

In February 2012 the private company Circle took over entire operational control of Hinchingbrooke Hospital in Cambridge. In January 2015 they announced that they were pulling out of the contract as they weren't getting adequate returns. Privatisation of management is also ongoing in a different way with the Department of Health awarding contracts to some of the biggest management consultancies and accountancy firms. They will share in a £200m pot to offer 'failing' NHS hospitals strategic direction and temporary management. Deloitte, Ernst and Young and McKinsey are amongst those due to benefit.[15]

The Blood Service

In July 2013 the Government sold an 80 per cent stake in the state-owned blood products business Plasma Resources to Bain Capital for £200m.[16]

Private Finance Initiative (PFI)

Hospitals built under the private finance initiative where companies design, finance, build and operate services are an early example of privatisation. The cost of PFI is a continuing burden for many hospitals. In 2013/14, 9 out of the 15 most 'indebted' trusts had PFI schemes. PFI is now widely recognised as providing very poor value. Around a hundred

NHS hospitals have been built this way. The cost to the tax payer will be £80bn for hospitals that cost nearly £13bn to build.[17]

Section 75

Section 75 of the HSC Act 2012 has been described as the 'engine of privatisation' as it ensures that NHS contracts are opened up to the market. The regulations later attached to it state that CCGs must put all services out to tender unless they can prove the service could only be provided by one particular provider.[18] The effect has been to provide many more opportunities for the private sector and charities to bid to run NHS services.[19]

Any Qualified Provider (AQP)

This policy introduced competition across a huge range of community health care. Private companies and charities can apply to join a list of approved health providers alongside existing NHS services. Each provider, including existing NHS services, will be paid according to how many NHS patients choose their service. There are now 39 community health services for which AQP can be used by commissioning bodies to award contracts, including areas such as adult hearing services, continuing care for adults and children, dermatology, pain services, endoscopy and ophthalmology.[20]

2. The impact of the NHS reforms

Advances in NHS care 'going into reverse'

Two health think tanks claim that improvements in recent years to vital NHS services such as GP consultations, planned surgery and treatment in A&E – in terms of both quality and access – are 'starting to go into reverse'.[21] Research by the Nuffield Trust and the Health Foundation published by *Pulse*

Today found:

- Hospital A&E units missed the NHS target of treating and either admitting or discharging 95 per cent of A&E patients within four hours for over a year in 2013-14.
- The number of patients experiencing a 'trolley wait', a delay of at least four hours between the decision to admit them at A&E and their arrival on a ward, rose from 93,905 in 2010-11, to 167,941 in 2013-14 – an increase of 79 per cent.
- One in ten patients had to wait more than the supposed 18-week maximum for planned treatment, mainly elective surgery such as cataract removal, in 2014.
- Patients are waiting four days longer for such treatment than they did in 2010.
- Waiting times for mental health patients to be assessed by a specialist have risen by a third, and in 2013 such patients waited almost twice as long to be assessed as people with physical ailments.
- The number of nurses working in psychiatric hospitals has fallen by 13 per cent since 2010, despite a 17 per cent rise in the number of patients detained for treatment.

The researchers also found that patients are finding it harder to get a GP appointment and 250,000 fewer older people now receive free social care services.

Spending on management consultancy in the NHS doubles in four years

In December 2014, Professor David Oliver, Visiting Professor in the School of Community and Health Sciences at City University, writing in the *BMJ* noted that spending on management consultants had more than doubled from £313m to £640m per year between 2010 and 2014, even though the coalition vowed to clamp down on the practice. The figures were obtained through a Freedom of Information request made by Professor Oliver.

In his article, Professor Oliver likened management consultants to 'racketeers' profiteering from 'times of chaos'. He warned that the staggering fees charged were hurting the health services. The investigation found that many senior partners in the consultancy firms charge £3000-£4000 a day – the amount that a senior doctor earns in two weeks. Professor Oliver singled out examples including Barts and the Royal London Hospitals, which spent £935,000 on advice from Global Titanium Solutions, about twice the combined salary of the trust's chief executive, chairman, and finance director; and West Dorset Clinical Commissioning Group, which is currently spending £2.7m with McKinsey for a 'strategic review'. He warned that consultancy firms 'are unaccountable and can walk away from bad or damaging advice with no consequences', adding, 'I have lost count of the number of reports that model drastic reductions in urgent activity or cost, based on no credible peer reviewed evidence'.[22]

Top cancer doctor's damning letter: 'NHS cuts will kill patients'
The Mirror revealed that some of the country's leading neurosurgeons and doctors were warning that savage cuts are putting cancer patients' lives at risk.[23] Lead consultant neurosurgeon Matthias Radatz said 'The changes last year were draconian and patients who wait for radiosurgery have been left totally in limbo. 'To the layman it's appalling. To the expert it's appalling.' In a damning letter to NHS bosses, he and other experts expressed their frustration and anger at the planned closure of 18 specialist centres to treat victims of brain cancer. They blamed the coalition changes to the NHS and the plan to cut £20bn from the NHS budget by 2015.

Cancer care commissioning is in chaos since NHS reorganisation, says leading charity

The government's reorganisation of the NHS in England has caused chaos in the commissioning of cancer care services, [24] which now needs radical change to be made fit for purpose, says a report from Cancer Research UK.[25]

The charity said that confused structures, unclear account-ability, and loss of national oversight, combined with in-sufficient funding, threatened to reverse hard won gains in survival rates among people with cancer. Harpal Kumar, the charity's chief executive, said that cancer services were now at a 'tipping point', with staff fighting to keep them viable in a context of flat-lined budgets and rising demand from patients.

Outsourcing: same job, same hours, same clients, less pay

An analysis by the Smith Institute think tank has shown that private companies taking over outsourced public sector contracts seek to drive down wage costs.[26] The report showed that low paid workers have been disproportionately affected, in one case losing up to 40 per cent of take home pay after being transferred to new employers. A further example involved the provision of a former NHS-run disability care service.[27] Large cuts to local government budgets meant that the only way to provide any service at all at the new lower contract values was for the provider to radically drive down employee terms and conditions. The main impact of outsourcing is therefore not to raise quality but to drive down wages.

NHS Trusts focusing more on private patient income to make up revenue gaps

NHS Trusts are placing a greater emphasis on the income they can receive from private patients, as a result of the decision to allow them to raise up to 49 per cent of their revenue from private treatment – up from 2 per cent – which was part of the NHS reforms in 2012. Some trusts have more than doubled the amount of income they receive from private work in the last two years.[28]

The patients who can't leave hospital – as no one will make a profit

Some patients who are otherwise fit to be discharged are unable to leave hospital as the private providers who are there to provide social care are unwilling to provide a care package which would enable the patient to return home, as it is not profitable for them to do so. The number of patients who suffer a 'Delayed Transfer Of Care' (DTOC, commonly termed 'bedblocking') is currently at its highest ever recorded level – in January 2015 figures showed that delayed discharges had risen by a third when compared to the same period a year earlier, with 62,000 'bed days' lost in the preceding month.[29]

Safety concerns over private sector surgery

The series of botched cataract removals carried out by a private clinic in Somerset which was given NHS work has raised concerns about the proportion of eye procedures done by the private sector, with one in every ten NHS cataract operations now being done by private health providers. The Royal National Institute of Blind People (RNIB) said that the need to guarantee patient safety in the private sector had become a 'key concern'.[30]

GP-led local NHS bodies forced to put health services out to tender

Research by *Health Service Journal* shows that 29.1 per cent of the leaders of 93 clinical commissioning groups (CCG) which responded to a survey said they had opened up, or were opening up, services to competition which they would not have done if they were not concerned about the impact of new rules contained in the controversial HSC Act. They included contracts for out-of-hours GP care, older people's services, audiology, ultrasound and podiatry.[31] In 2012, the health secretary Andrew Lansley wrote to all the 211 CCGs pledging unequivocally that they individually would be able to decide, rather than ministers or the NHS regulator, Monitor, when to put contracts out to tender.[32] But the same *HSJ* found that 20 per cent of CCGs had encountered a challenge under the new competition rules to a decision they had taken about the commissioning of services, while 57 per cent had experienced 'informal challenge or questioning'. In addition, 65 per cent of the 103 bosses of the 93 CCGs said that they had incurred extra costs related to commissioning as a result of the regulations, while 36 per cent said they had hampered plans for local hospitals to merge or become foundation trusts.

3. The views of NHS staff and users

The vast majority of NHS staff say reform had negative impact

Only 5 per cent of health professionals in a survey by Dods said that there was a positive impact for the NHS changes. Of the 3,628 NHS staff questioned many believe that improving patient care now comes second to making savings. 'Money is a prime concern with only 2 per cent saying their organisation had sufficient financial resource and 71 per cent disagreeing with the idea that they have enough budgetary support to support their organisation.'[33]

Two in five fear the NHS will soon cease to be free

More than two out of five people fear the NHS will cease to be a free service over the next twenty years. 44 per cent said it was unlikely and 37 per cent thought it was likely to be the case. The findings came from a survey of 1,030 adults in England by pollsters Populus and were publised shortly after several think tanks, groups of health professionals and ex-Labour health minister Lord Warner had proposed that the NHS should introduce charges, notably for visiting GPs, as a way of reducing the burden on the taxpayer.[34]

85 per cent of GPs believe the NHS will be privatised within ten years

Almost 85 per cent of GPs believe the NHS will be privatised within ten years, with 45 per cent predicting it will occur within five years, a survey of 1,137 NHS staff has revealed. The survey, conducted by Cogora, which publishes *Pulse*, also revealed that GPs felt less engaged in the CCG decision-making than practice managers. It found that 91 per cent of GPs felt the reforms resulted in more work, while 97 per cent of practice managers believe workload had increased. The survey questioned 548 GPs, 418 nurses and 171 practice managers. It found that exactly half of practice managers felt that privatisation will happen within seven years, compared with 45 per cent of GPs. Only 14 per cent of GPs and 11 per cent of practice managers felt that privatisation will not occur in the next ten years.[35]

Practice survey reveals just one fifth of GPs expect their practice to survive

Only a fifth of GPs expect their practice to still exist in ten years, according to devastating results of a wide-ranging survey of practice staff on the future of general practice published by the GP magazine *Pulse*.[36] The poll was initiated locally by a practice manager in Oxford and ended up being cascaded right across England, receiving over 2,700 responses, three-quarters of which were from GPs. The final results showed only 20 per cent of respondents were confident their practice would exist in 10 years, while a third said the exact opposite.

Almost all the respondents – 97 per cent – agreed their practice was 'experiencing an ever increasing and unsustainable pressure of work', while 68 per cent told an *HSJ* poll their referral rate was likely to increase in order to cope with increased demands on general practice.

Four-fifths of respondents said they believed one or more GPs in their practice was suffering from 'burnout'.[37]

Junior doctors raise patient care concerns

Most junior doctors do not feel they have enough time to care for patients, according to a new poll. Of the 1,000 training medics polled by the Medical Protection Society, 70 per cent said they feel as though they do not have enough time to give patients the care they need.[38] And half said that they had concerns about quality of care in their workplace. Meanwhile, 82 per cent said they struggled with long hours in the last year, and almost two-thirds said they had difficulty with heavy workloads.

Keep politics out of NHS, says poll

The vast majority of the public believe that MPs play political football with the NHS, a new poll suggests, as doctors called for the government's controversial reforms of the NHS to be scrapped. Almost three-quarters of people – 73 per cent – told the pollsters that political parties design health policy to win votes rather than do what is best for the health service.[39] Meanwhile, the questionnaire of 2,000 people from across Britain shows that two in three believe the NHS should manage itself without the involvement of politicians. Only one in three said that parliament should set targets for the health service.

Information and Campaigning: some starting points

Selected Campaigning Organisations and Parties

Centre for Health and Public Interest: research and reports on public health politics, http://chpi.org.uk/reports/ e.g.: Calum Paton, *At what cost? Paying the price for the market in the English NHS.* http://chpi.org.uk/; twitter @CHPIthinktank.

Doctors for the NHS (NHS Consultants Association): campaigning against privatisation; briefings, policy research. http://www.nhsca.org.uk/.

Green Party: Maintain a publicly funded, publicly provided health service, and oppose NHS privatisation and treating health care as a market. http://greenparty.org.uk/values/nhs-2010/nhs-detail.html; twitter @TheGreenParty.

Keep Our NHS Public: campaigns for a publicly funded, publicly delivered and publicly accountable NHS; a national organisation with local groups. www.keepournhspublic.com; twitter @keepnhspublic.

London Health Emergency: news, analysis, campaigns. See especially John Lister, *Briefings for Cynical Commissioning Groups,* 2014. http://www.healthemergency.org.uk/pdf/CynicalCommissioningGroups1.pdf http//www.healthemergency.org.uk; twitter @JohnRLister.

Medsin: works amongst students on global and local health issues. http://www.medsin.org/; twitter @medsinuk.

National Health Action Party: campaigns for a publicly funded, publicly delivered and publicly accountable NHS. http://nhap.org/our-policies-1/. http://www.nationalhealthaction.org.uk; twitter @NHAparty.

NHS Support Federation: campaigns to improve and protect the NHS in keeping with its founding principles. Maps, statistics, news. http://www.nhscampaign.org; twitter @nhs_supporters.

OpenDemocracy: 'free thinking for the world'. See especially: 'OurNHS',working for a decent National Health Service in England. http://www.opendemocracy.net/ournhs/about; twitter @OurNHS_oD.

People vs. PFI: campaign against PFI; 'private interests make profit through the Private Finance Initiative – quietly killing off our public services.' http://www.peoplevspfi.org.uk/.

People's vote for the NHS: 'we have to save the NHS from the greed & corruption of private companies. NHS for people, not profit.' http://999callfornhs.org.uk; http://www.peoplesvotefornhs.org.uk/.

Spinwatch: lobbies for transparency, and seeks to uncover commercial lobbies, PR and propaganda. http://www.spinwatch.org/; twitter @Spinwatch.

UNISON Health Care: campaigns on policies, cuts, pay, pensions, and more. http://www.unison.org.uk/at-work/health-care/; twitter @ourNHS.

Unite the Union: runs a Save our NHS campaign http://www.unitetheunion.org/how-we-help/list-of-sectors/healthsector/healthsectorcampaigns/unite4ournhs/ and has published a very useful and informative *Guide to NHS Privatisation*: http://www.unitetheunion.org/uploaded/

documents/GuideToNHSPrivatisation11-10734.pdf.
http://www.unitetheunion.org; twitter @unitetheunion.

Further Reading

Jacky Davis & Raymond Tallis – editors, *NHS SOS: how the NHS was betrayed – and how we can save it*, Oneworld, 2013.

Colin Leys & Stewart Player, *The Plot against the NHS*, Merlin Press, 2011.
—, *Confuse and Conceal*, Merlin Press, 2008.

John Lister, *Health Policy Reform: Global Health versus Private Profit*, Libri Publishing, 2013.
—, *The NHS After 60 – For patients or profits?* Libri, 2008.
People's Inquiry into London's NHS, http://www.
peoplesinquiry.org/pdf/NHSattheCrossroadsfulldoc.pdf.

Allyson M. Pollock, *The End of the NHS*, Verso, 2015.
—, *NHS plc: The Privatisation of Our Health Care*, Verso Books, 2004.

NHS England policy documents, for example *Five Year Forward View*, reveal certain future perspectives, http://www.england.nhs.uk/wp-content/uploads/2014/10/5yfv-web.pdf. Their website and that of other public bodies, are listed on pages viii-x.

Video

Sell off, Peter Bach, 2014
trailer: https://www.youtube.com/watch?v=wvUIobKvXJg

The Spirit of '45, Ken Loach, 2013
trailer: https://www.youtube.com/watch?v=_c86Gwsb5LY

Sicko, Michael Moore, 2007
trailer: https://www.youtube.com/watch?v=UReMPrjMT9E

Spinwatch Health Industry Lobbying Tour
https://www.youtube.com/watch?v=WDj-1D6U0LU

Taking Action

Those who want to join the fight to save the NHS are referred to the relevant chapter in *NHS SOS* (listed above): 'What you can do to save the NHS'.

Notes

Introduction

1. McKee M. 2012 'Does anyone understand the government's plan for the NHS?' *BMJ* 2012;344:e399.

2. Lansley A. 2012. 'Why legislation is necessary for my health reforms.' *BMJ* 2012;344:e789.

3. Klein R. 2013. 'Sleepwalking into a political fiasco.' *Health Economics, Policy and Law* 2013;8(02):237-42.

4. R v Campell. EWCA Crim 726, [2006] 2 Cr App R (S) 626 [2006].

5. R (on the application of the DPP) v South East Surrey Youth Court (Ghanbari ip. EWHC 2929 (Admin), [2006] 2 All ER 444. [2005].

6. King A, Crewe I. 2013. *The Blunders of Our Governments*. London: Oneworld Publications.

7. Himmelstein DU, Thorne D, Warren E, Woolhandler S. 2009. 'Medical bankruptcy in the United States, 2007: results of a national study.' *Am J Med* 2009;122(8):741-6.

8. Reynolds L, McKee M. 2012. 'Opening the oyster: the 2010-11 NHS reforms in England.' *Clin Med* 2012;12(2):128-32.

9. Letwin O. 1988. *Privatising the world*. London: Cassell.

10. Reynolds L, McKee M. 2012. 'GP commissioning and the NHS reforms: what lies behind the hard sell?' *J R Soc Med* 2012;105(1):7-10.

11. van Ginneken E, Groenewegen PP, McKee M. 2012 'Personal healthcare budgets: what can England learn from the Netherlands?' *BMJ* 2012;344:e1383.

12. Carroll L. 2012. *Alice's adventures in Wonderland and Through the looking glass*. London: Penguin.

13. Peedell C. 2011. 'Further privatisation is inevitable under the proposed NHS reforms', *BMJ* 2011;342:d2996.

14. McKee M. 2013. The future of England's healthcare lies in the hands of competition lawyers. *BMJ* 2013;346:f1733.

15. Voltaire. 1997. *Candide*. London: Penguin.

16. Travis A. 2013. 'Serious Fraud Office launches inquiry into G4S and Serco overcharging claims'. *Guardian* 2013;http://www.theguardian.com/law/2013/nov/04/serious-fraud-office-inquiry-g4s-serco-overcharging.

17. Iacobucci G. 2014. 'Serco plans to pull out of clinical service provision in the UK.' *BMJ* 2014;349:g5248.

18. Deith J. 2014. 'Serco penalised by pound 81,000 a month over failings in Suffolk contract.' *BMJ* 2014;348:g1167.

19. Rameesh R. 2012. 'NHS lab failings followed Serco-led takeover.' *Guardian* 2012;http://www.theguardian.com/society/2012/sep/30/pathology-labs-takeover-failures.

20. O'Dowd A. 2013. 'MPs condemn Serco for substandard out of hours service in Cornwall.' *BMJ* 2013;347:f4479.

21. Krachler N, Greer I. 2014. 'When does marketisation lead to privatisation? Profit-making in English health services after the 2012 Health and Social Care Act.' *Soc Sci Med* 2014;124C:215-23.

22. Loewenstein A. 2014. 'Serco is failing, but is kept afloat thanks to Australia's refugee policy.' *Guardian* 2014;http://www.theguardian.com/commentisfree/2014/nov/11/serco-is-failing-but-is-maintained-afloat-thanks-to-australias-refugee-policy.

23. McKee M, Karanikolos M, Belcher P, Stuckler D. 2012 'Austerity: a failed experiment on the people of Europe.' *Clin Med* 2012;12(4):346-50.

24. Tallis R, Davis J. 2013. *NHS SOS: how the NHS was betrayed - and how we can save it.* London: Oneworld Publications.

25. McSmith A. Letwin. 2004. 'NHS will not exist under Tories'. *The Independent* 2004;http://www.independent.co.uk/life-style/health-and-families/health-news/letwin-nhs-will-not-exist-under-tories-6168295.html.

26. Meikle J. 2014. 'NHS still struggling to cope with extra patients as funding deal agreed.' *Guardian* 2014;http://www.theguardian.com/society/2014/dec/19/nhs-staff-strikes-new-year-pay-hospitals.

27. Jarman H. 2014. 'Public health and the Transatlantic trade and investment partnership.' *European Journal of Public Health* 2014;24(2):181-81.

28. Desai M, Nolte E, Karanikolos M, Khoshaba B, McKee M. 2011. 'Measuring NHS performance 1990-2009 using amenable mortality: interpret with care.' *J R Soc Med* 2011;104(9):370-9.

29. Ingleby D, McKee M, Mladovsky P, Rechel B. 2012. 'How the NHS measures up to other health systems.' *BMJ* 2012;344:e1079.

30. Figueras J, McKee M. 2012 *Health systems, health, wealth and societal well-being : assessing the case for investing in health systems.* Maidenhead: McGraw-Hill Open University Press.

31. McKee M, Basu S, Stuckler D. 2012. 'Health systems, health and wealth: the argument for investment applies now more than ever.' *Soc Sci Med* 2012;74(5):684-7.

32. Reeves A, Basu S, McKee M, Meissner C, Stuckler D. 2013. 'Does investment in the health sector promote or inhibit economic growth?' *Global Health* 2013;9:43.

33. Arrow KJ. 1963. Uncertainty and the welfare economics of medical care.

The American economic review 1963:941-73.

34. Sinclair U. 1994. 'I, candidate for governor, and how I got licked.' Berkeley: University of California Press.

35. Meikle J. 2013 'Jeremy Hunt loses appeal as Lewisham hospital cuts ruled illegal.' Guardian 2013;http://www.theguardian.com/society/2013/oct/29/lewisham-hospital-jeremy-hunt-unlawful.

Chapter I

1   Giles, C. 2014. Britain and the cuts: Blow for Cameron as UK faces deeper cuts, Financial Times, 10 November, http://www.ft.com/cms/s/2/5426fc12-6346-11e4-8a63-00144feabdc0.html#axzz3IgRavh6t.

2   Donnelly L. 2014. 'Dozens of maternity and A&E units shut', Daily Telegraph, 26 October, http://www.telegraph.co.uk/journalists/laura-donnelly/11184764/Dozens-of-maternity-and-AandE-units-shut.html.

3   Ross T. 2012. Downing Street 'does not want Andrew Lansley 'taken out and shot', Daily Telegraph, 7 February, http://www.telegraph.co.uk/health/healthnews/9066483/Downing-Street-does-not-want-Andrew-Lansley-taken-out-and-shot.html.

4   Calkin S. 2013. 'Bournemouth and Poole merger is blocked', Health Service Journal, 17 October: http://www.hsj.co.uk/5064392.article?WT.tsrc=Email&WT.mc_id=EditEmailStory&referrer=e94.

5   Calkin S. 2013b. Concern over Monitor's Bristol 'merger' decision, Health Service Journal, 24 September, http://www.hsj.co.uk/news/commissioning/concern-over-monitors-bristol-merger-decision/5063548.article?blocktitle=News&contentID=8805.

6   http://stopttip.net/ttip-and-its-impact-on-the-nhs-and-health/.

7   According to his own answer on BBC's Question Time programme: BBC1, 16 October, 2014.

8   Smyth C, 2014. 'NHS reforms our worst mistake, Tories admit', The Times, 13 October, http://www.thetimes.co.uk/tto/news/politics/article4234883.ece.

9   http://www.theguardian.com/society/2014/jun/21/nhs-control-given-away-tory-minister.

10   Regular updates on the progress of privatisation can be found at the NHS for Sale website run by the NHS Support Federation http://www.nhsforsale.info/privatisation-list.html.

11   Molloy, C. 2014. 'The billions of wasted NHS cash no-one wants to mention', Our NHS, 10 October 2014 https://www.opendemocracy.net/ournhs/caroline-molloy/billions-of-wasted-nhs-cash-noone-wants-to-mention.

12 Stevenson A. 2014. 'It's official: No-one knows who is in charge of the NHS', www.politics.co.uk 10 November, http://www.politics.co.uk/news/2014/11/10/it-s-official-no-one-knows-who-is-in-charge-of-the-nhs.

13 http://www.publications.parliament.uk/pa/cm201415/cmselect/cmpubadm/110/110.pdf.

14 http://www.theguardian.com/society/2013/dec/21/nhs-service-jeremy-hunt-malcolm-grant.

15 Lintern S. 2014. Exclusive: NHS England primary care decisions 'unlawful', High Court rules, *HSJ*, 24 November. http://www.hsj.co.uk/news/exclusive-nhs-england-primary-care-decisions-unlawful-high-court-rules/5077054.article?blocktitle=News&contentID=8805#.VHNp0o1ybxk.

16 http://www.britishkidney-pa.co.uk/images/stories/news_images/BKPA_briefing_on_commissioning_of_dialysis_services_v1.docx.

17 NHS Confederation. 2014. 'Tough times, tough choices, Being open and honest about NHS finance', http://www.nhsconfed.org/~/media/Confederation/Files/Publications/Documents/Tough-times-open-honest-report.pdf.

18 Crawford, R., Emmerson, C., and Keynes, S. 2014. 'Public finances: risks on tax, bigger risks on spending?' (In *The IFS Green Budget: February 2014*), Institute of Fiscal Studies, London, http://www.ifs.org.uk/budgets/gb2014/gb2014_ch2.pdf.

19 The King's Fund's Barker Commission report (2014:20) points out that from 1948-1999 the average increase in real terms was just 3 per cent per year, while the ten years from 2000 saw increases from 6-7 per cent.

20 In Mid Staffs cuts in staffing levels were used as a main tool to force down spending and present an appearance of balanced books to the foundation trust regulator, Monitor, and achieve foundation status early in 2008 – at the expense of plunging standards of patient care, which were not picked up until later; *Metro*, 6 February, 2013.

21 Campbell D. 2014. 'NHS staff shortages pose risk to patients, warns watchdog', *The Guardian*, 17 October; http://www.theguardian.com/society/2014/oct/17/nhs-staff-shortages-risk-patients-cqc-report.

22 In a landmark report by management consultants McKinsey – many consider this report as inadequate, ill-conceived and misleading. Department of Health, 2010, McKinsey report on the fiscal future of the NHS, 2 June 2010, http://webarchive.nationalarchives.gov.uk/+/www.dh.gov.uk/en/FreedomOfInformation/Freedomofinformationpublicationschemefeedback/FOIreleases/DH_116520.

23 Kurunmäki, L., Miller, P. 2011. 'The Failure of a Failure Regime: From

Insolvency to De-Authorisation for NHS Foundation Trusts', LSE Centre for Analysis of Risk and Regulation, Discussion Paper No: 67, http://www.lse.ac.uk/accounting/facultyAndStaff/profiles/CARR per cent20DP per cent20Peter per cent20and per cent20Liisa.pdf.

24 http://www.england.nhs.uk/ourwork/futurenhs/.

25 Press Association. 2014. 'Fund NHS properly or charge for hospital beds, says senior executive', The Guardian 7 October; http://www.theguardian.com/society/2014/oct/07/fund-nhs-properly-or-charge-for-hospital-beds-says-senior-executive.

26 Barker, K. 2014. A new settlement for health and social care, The Barker Commission report, King's Fund, London available: http://www.kingsfund.org.uk/publications/new-settlement-health-and-social-care

27 Warner N, O'Sullivan J (2014) Solving the NHS care and cash crisis: Routes to health and care renewal, Reform, available http://www.reform.co.uk/content/32643/research/health/solving_the_nhs_care_and_cash_crisis.

28 Stevenson A. 2014. 'Ed Miliband: We'll tax the rich to heal the sick', 23 September, http://www.politics.co.uk/news/2014/09/23/ed-miliband-well-tax-the-rich-to-heal-the-poor.

29 http://www.nhshistory.net/chapter per cent207.htm.

30 The Guardian, 26 October 1998.

31 HSJ, 1 June 1995.

32 HSJ, 22 August 1996.

33 Department of Health Press Release, 7 April 1998.

34 'The Tory attempt to use private money to build hospitals has failed to deliver. Labour will overcome the problems that have plagued the Private Finance Initiative, end the delays, sort out the confusion and develop new forms of public/private partnership that work better and protect the interests of the NHS. Labour Manifesto, 1997, available http://www.labour-party.org.uk/manifestos/1997/1997-labour-manifesto.shtml.

35 Speech from Baroness Jay moving the Bill: http://hansard.millbanksystems.com/lords/1997/jun/03/national-health-service-private-finance.

36 BBC News. 2014. Sherwood Forest Hospitals Trust's PFI bill revealed, 16 October; http://www.bbc.co.uk/news/uk-england-nottinghamshire-29636743.

37 Lister J. 2013. 'Pure Financial Incompetence, The Heavy price of PFI in the NHS in Eastern Region', UNISON Eastern Region, http://www.healthemergency.org.uk/pdf/PureFinancialIncompetence.pdf.

38 Trust Special Administrator. 2014. 'Securing sustainable NHS services:

the Trust Special Administrator's report on South London Healthcare NHS Trust and the NHS in south east London; (Vol. 1, p. 15ff; https://www.gov.uk/government/uploads/system/uploads/attachment_data/file/213341/TSA-VOL-1.pdf.

39 One unfortunate side effect of this successful challenge was that there has still never been a proper external appraisal of the viability of the TSA's proposals and their total cost.

40 http://www.midstaffspublicinquiry.com/.

41 This is discussed in greater detail in Chapter 4.

42 *Yorkshire Post.* 2013. 'Anger over £6m taxpayer bill for NHS advisors', 15 March, http://www.yorkshirepost.co.uk/news/main-topics/general-news/exclusive-anger-over-6m-taxpayer-bill-for-nhs-advisors-1-5501372.

43 This is discussed in greater detail in Chapter 4.

44 Department of Health. 2013. 'Investment in mental health in 2011 to 2012: working age adults and older adults'; https://www.gov.uk/government/publications/investment-in-mental-health-in-2011-to-2012-working-age-adults-and-older-adults.

45 Large, Z. 2014. 'Major failings' in CAMHS Tier Four services, a new review reveals, YoungMinds, July available http://www.youngminds.org.uk/news/blog/2137_major_failings_in_camhs_tier_four_services_a_new_review_reveals.

46 http://www.nhsconfed.org/Networks/MentalHealth/LatestNews/Pages/Nick_Clegg_launches_action_plan.aspx.

47 'The A&E departments at Ealing and Charing Cross hospitals must be sustained until further work to inform a final decision on the future of these two local hospitals has been completed and the alternative services that will provide a safe, high quality urgent emergency care system for local residents are in place.' (p. 6 of IRP report), available: https://www.gov.uk/government/uploads/system/uploads/attachment_data/file/358743/000_LNW_report_13.09.13.pdf.

48 This and the following two paragraphs are based on information in Costly Savings, a report researched by John Lister for East Midlands Region of UNISON in spring 2014.

49 Baker, K. 2014. 'Virgin boss Sir Richard Branson bids to take over cancer and end of life care in NHS privatisation deal worth £1.2bn', Mail Online, 6 November http://www.dailymail.co.uk/news/article-2823946/Sir-Richard-Branson-bids-NHS-privatisation-deal-worth-1-2billion.html#ixzz3N7k6F3f9.

50 BBC News. 2014. 'Extreme worry' over NHS Kernow £75m procurement plans', 25 June: http://www.bbc.co.uk/news/uk-england-cornwall-28025139.

51 Watt, N. 2014. 'Income from private patients soars at NHS hospital trusts', *The Guardian* 19 August, available http://www.theguardian.com/society/2014/aug/19/private-patient-income-soars-nhs-privatisation

52 Association of Directors of Adult Social Services. 2013. 'Social care funding: 'a bleak outlook is getting bleaker', 6 May; http://www.adass.org.uk/index.php?option=com_content&id=914&Itemid=489.

53 Audit Commission. 2013. 'Social care for older people Using data from the VFM Profiles', July http://www.audit-commission.gov.uk/2013/07/audit-commission-analyses-cost-of-social-care-for-older-people-in-a-value-for-money-briefing/.

54 Thomson A, Sylvester R. 2014. 'This is going to hurt: it's patients who pay as money runs out', *The Times*, 13 October, http://www.thetimes.co.uk/tto/health/news/article4234741.ece https://nhsreality.wordpress.com/2014/10/13/this-is-going-to-hurt-its-patients-who-pay-as-money-runs-out/).

55 Lister J. 2014. 'Behind the Smoke and Mirrors, neither Hinchingbrooke nor Circle are what they seem', UNISON Eastern Region; http://www.unisoneastern.org.uk/assets/library/document/s/original/smoke_and_mirrors.pdf.

56 Available http://www.nhsstaffsurveys.com/Caches/Files/NHS_staff_survey_2013_RQQ_full.pdf.

57 Maude F., Lamb N. 2014. Mutuals in Health: Pathfinder Programme, Letter to foundation trusts, 24 July, available: https://www.gov.uk/government/uploads/system/uploads/attachment_data/file/343507/Letter_to_Foundation_Trusts_and_NHS_Trusts.pdf.

58 Department of Health. 2014. Application pack: https://www.gov.uk/government/uploads/system/uploads/attachment_data/file/343503/Mutuals_in_health_pathfinder_programme_application_pack.pdf.

59 See the response from UNISON Eastern Region to the various plans for hiving off community health services, available http://www.healthemergency.org.uk/workingwu/TCS4pager.pdf.

60 http://www.kingsfund.org.uk/blog/2014/07/staff-led-nhs-improving-patient-care-engaging-staff-and-devolving-decision-making.

61 Lister J. 2007. *Fragmenting the NHS*, UNISON Oxfordshire Health Branch; http://www.healthemergency.org.uk/workingwu/SocialEnterprisepamphlet.pdf.

62 Landale J. 2011. Plans to outsource public services 'scaled back', BBC News, 3 May, http://www.bbc.co.uk/news/uk-politics-13273932.

63 Estimated at £1m.

64 BBC News. 2014. 'Jarrow March' ends in pro-NHS rally in London, 6 September, http://www.bbc.co.uk/news/uk-england-29094093.

65 Stoye G. 2013. 'Public payment and private provision: the changing
    landscape of healthcare in the 2000s', IFS May 2013, available http://
    www.nuffieldtrust.org.uk/publications/public-payment-private-
    provision-2000s.
66 http://www.england.nhs.uk/wp-content/uploads/2014/10/5yfv-web.pdf.

Chapter 2

1   BMJ2011;342:d566.
2   It also uses data from the Organisation for Economic Co-operation
    and Development and from the World Health Organisation. No one
    challenges its credentials.
3   http://www.commonwealthfund.org/publications/fund-reports/2014/jun/
    mirror-mirror.
4   BMJ2014;348:g3063.
5   http://www.telegraph.co.uk/health/10550335/UK-has-fewer-doctors-per-
    person-than-Bulgaria-and-Estonia.html.
6   EF http://www.telegraph.co.uk/health/healthnews/10768844/Hospital-
    bed-shortage-exposed.html.
7   www.bmj.com/content/348/bmj.g3129.
8   O'Dowd A. Balance between GP and hospital doctor numbers may
    need to shift, says new NHS chief. BMJ2014;348:g3037.
9   BMJ2014;348:g3129.
10 http://www.pulsetoday.co.uk/political/political-news/dh-to-hand-over-
    22bn-underspend-to-treasury/20004042.article#.VF9UTWlgGK1.
11 http://news.rapgenius.com/Noam-chomsky-the-state-corporate-
    complex-a-threat-to-freedom-and-survival-annotated#.
12 http://www.reform.co.uk/resources/0000/1069/The_cost_of_our_health__
    the_role_of_charging_in_healthcare.pdf.
13 http://www.theguardian.com/commentisfree/2014/mar/31/10-pounds-
    each-save-nhs.
14 BMJ2014;348:g3498.
15 Scotland, Wales and Northern Ireland have not followed the English
    NHS down the path of marketisation. The prospect of a marketised NHS
    being imported across the border into Scotland was used to encourage
    a 'yes' vote for independence in the Scots referendum.
16 http://www.publications.parliament.uk/pa/cm200910/cmselect/
    cmhealth/268/26803.htm.
17 BMJ2012;344:e2868.
18 BMJ2013;347:f5550.
19 BMJ2013;347:f5550.

20 BMJ2013;347:f5550.

21 ref http://www.bmj.com/content/347/bmj.f6246.

22 BMJ2013;347:f5862.

23 BMJ2013;346:f1733.

24 http://www.pulsetoday.co.uk/commissioning/commissioning-topics/
    ccgs/first-ccgs-under-investigation-for-breach-of-competition-
    regulations/20004715.article#.VJLtIPmsWHk.

25 In New Zealand an experiment in getting rid of the purchaser/provider
    split resulted in improved care for patients and a reduced demand
    on hospital services. GPs and consultants came together to improve
    decision making instead of competing with each other for funds.
    BMJ2013;347:f5503.

26 BMJ2014;349:g4515.

27 A Comres poll in 2014 reported that 60 per cent of those who expressed
    an opinion would be prepared to pay more income tax if it was ring-
    fenced for the NHS, a sign of the high value the public places on the
    service. http://www.theguardian.com/society/2014/aug/15/voters-tax-
    fund-nhs-poll.

Chapter 3

1 http://www.telegraph.co.uk/news/politics/6060421/David-Cameron-the-
   NHS-is-safe-under-the-Conservatives.html.

2 http://www.england.nhs.uk/ourwork/gov/choiceandcompetition/.

3 For more details of the early NHS see: Lister J. 2008. *The NHS After 60:
   for Patients or Profits?* Faringdon: Libri Publishing.

4 'What lies beneath?' *HealthInvestor,* 8 September 2010.

5 http://www.margaretthatcher.org/document/107565.

6 https://www.thegazette.co.uk/London/issue/50154/supplement/1.

7 Mathiason N, 2000. 'Labour gets into bed with private medicine', *The
   Observer* 19 November, http://www.theguardian.com/society/2000/
   nov/19/socialcare.policy.

8 http://www.mirror.co.uk/news/uk-news/patients-occupy-clinic-save-
   david-3417922;
   http://www.bbc.com/news/uk-england-stoke-staffordshire-28972225.

9 Attached to an article: 'Figures reveal decline in use of electronic
   referral system that allows patients to choose location of an
   outpatient appointment' Nicholas Watt, 24 November 2013 , http://
   www.theguardian.com/society/2013/nov/24/patient-choice-nhs-going-
   backwards-labour.

10 http://www.dailymail.co.uk/news/article-2673477/EXCLUSIVE-GPs-fail-

spot-cancer-named-shamed-Health-Secretary-tells-Mail-Sunday-radical-new-policy-crack-doctors-miss-vital-diagnosis.html#ixzz3NcMkOv53.

11 10 December 2014.

12 BMJ2014;348:g2274.

13 http://www.theguardian.com/society/2013/dec/28/sexual-health-clinics-doctors-fear-future-private?CMP=twt_gu.

14 http://www.hsj.co.uk/5063236.article?WT.mc_id=EditEmailStory&referrer=e2.

15 Paton, Calum. 2014. 'At what cost? Paying the price for the market in the English NHS' CHPI, http://chpi.org.uk/reports/.

16 https: //abetternhs.wordpress.com/2011/09/29/point/.

Chapter 4

1 Speech, July 2010, http://www.networks.nhs.uk/nhs-networks/qipp-network/news/andrew-lansleys-speech-on-an-nhs-driven-by-outcomes.

2 Letter to UK GPs, 16 February 2012.

3 Quoted by Tomlinson, J. 2011. *Betrayal of the NHS must end, it's time for doctors to fight back*, A Better NHS blog, 24 June, available. https://abetternhs.wordpress.com/2013/06/24/betrayal/.

4 http://www.hsj.co.uk/comment/prime-provider-contracts-are-a-solution-for-the-nhs-not-a-problem ; Corrigan P, Laitner S. 2012. *The Accountable Lead Provider*, rightcare.nhs.uk http://www.rightcare.nhs.uk/downloads/Rightcare_Casebook_accountable_lead_provider_Aug2012.pdf.

5 Iacobucci G. 2011. Just 5 per cent of GPs on commissioning group boards faced contested election, *Pulse* 28 September, available http://www.pulsetoday.co.uk/just-5-of-gps-on-commissioning-group-boards-faced-contested-election/12779846.article#.VKFh6DpAGg

6 http://www.nhscc.org/ccgs/.

7 http://www.gponline.com/exclusive-sharp-rise-gps-quitting-ccg-board-roles/article/1211757.

8 http://www.kingsfund.org.uk/sites/files/kf/field/field_publication_file/clinical-commissioning-groups-report-ings-fund-nuffield-jul13.pdf.

9 Kailash Chand, 'Jeremy Hunt should stop GP-bashing, or hospital referrals will skyrocket' http://www.theguardian.com/healthcare-network/2014/jun/30/jeremy-hunt-stop-gp-bashing.

10 http://www.ealingtoday.co.uk/shared/eaaeclosures002.htm?utm_content=buffer061ef&utm_medium=social&utm_source=twitter.com&utm_campaign=buffer; 'The Government is on a mission to bring it [the NHS] to its knees, so total privatisation can be hailed as the big rescuer': http://www.mirror.co.uk/news/uk-news/jeremy-hunt-michael-

gove-need-3778197# http://www.dailymail.co.uk/news/article-2673477/
EXCLUSIVE-GPs-fail-spot-cancer-named-shamed-Health-Secretary-tells-
Mail-Sunday-radical-new-policy-crack-doctors-miss-vital-diagnosis.
html.

11 http://www.bbc.co.uk/news/uk-politics-24362902.

12 http://www.bmj.com/content/347/bmj.f4351.

13 http://en.wikipedia.org/wiki/Nicholson_challenge.

14 http://webarchive.nationalarchives.gov.uk/+/
www.dh.gov.uk/en/FreedomOfInformation/
Freedomofinformationpublicationschemefeedback/FOIreleases/
DH_116520.

15 RCS. 2011. Procedures of Limited Clinical Value, a Briefing, available.
http://www.rcseng.ac.uk/publications/docs/rcs-briefing-procedures-of-
limited-clinical-value?searchterm=procedures+of+limited+clinical+val
ue.

16 http://www.england.nhs.uk/commissioning/wp-content/uploads/
sites/12/2014/11/nxt-steps-pc-cocomms.pdf.

17 http://www.unisoneastern.org.uk/assets/library/document/n/original/
newsletter_review_the_futurebedford_hospital_nhs_trust_.pdf.

18 http://blackpoolccg.nhs.uk/about-blackpool-ccg/who-we-are/our-
governing-body/.

19 http://www.nhsforsale.info/private-providers/private-provider-profiles-2/
virgin.html.

20 http://www.pulsetoday.co.uk/commissioning/conflict-of-interest-fears-
lead-virgin-to-take-over-gp-partnerships/20000663.article#.VF4avofCSng.

21 Nunns A. 2013. It is almost a year since the controversial Health and
Social Care Act was passed in March 2012, *Red Pepper* 18 February,
available. http://www.redpepper.org.uk/the-health-hurricane-a-year-of-
destruction-in-the-nhs/.

22 Full text available (page 7) http://www.healthemergency.org.uk/he-
issues/he71.pdf.

23 http://blackpoolccg.nhs.uk/wp-content/uploads/2014/09/Spire-Monitor-
Investigation-25.09.14.pdf.

24 http://www.hsj.co.uk/news/finance/regulator-rejects-private-hospitals-
complaint-against-ccgs/5075165.article#.VF-FSIfCSnh.

25 Calkin S. 2014. 'Devon presses ahead with procurement plans', *HSJ*, 7
November, available (£) http://www.hsj.co.uk/hsj-local/ccgs/nhs-north-
east-west-devon-ccg/new-devon-presses-ahead-with-procurement-
plans/5076567.article#.VHMrFo1ybxk.

26 Barnes S. 2014. Patient transport service fails to improve, HSJ 25
July, available. (£)http://www.hsj.co.uk/hsj-local/ccgs/nhs-west-

kent-ccg/patient-transport-service-fails-to-improve/5073302.article#.
VHMto41ybxk .

27 https://www.opendemocracy.net/ournhs/caroline-molloy-louise-irvine/
    stop-hospital-closure-clause.

28 http://www.newstatesman.com/politics/2014/01/clause-118-would-leave-
    no-hospital-england-safe.

29 http://www.unitetheunion.org/how-we-help/list-of-sectors/healthsector/
    healthsectorcampaigns/unite4ournhs/the-care-bill--clause-118/ .

30 http://www.nhscc.org.

31 http://www.nhscc.org/wp-content/uploads/2013/12/Letter-and-slide-
    clarifying-NHSCC-CA.pdf.

32 http://www.nhscc.org/about-us/whos-who/people/dr_johnny_marshall/.

33 http://www.neessexccg.nhs.uk/cms_useruploads/files/cc2h_full_
    business_care_for_board_nov_2014.pdf.

34 http://www.pulsetoday.co.uk/news/political-news/labour-to-remove-
    commissioning-powers-from-gps-for-vulnerable-patients/20007326.
    article#.VHIIPYvCSng.

35 http://www.england.nhs.uk/commissioning/wp-content/uploads/
    sites/12/2014/11/nxt-steps-pc-cocomms.pdf.

36 For the full story of the media's failure to challenge the legislation see
    NHS SOS.

37 http://www.gponline.com/gps-risk-losing-patient-trust-ccg-cuts-lmcs-
    warn/article/1183910.

38 http://www.hsj.co.uk/home/commissioning/clare-gerada-the-health-act-
    made-me-ill/5064376.article#.VF4KqIfCSng.

39 http://www.rcgp.org.uk/news/2013/october/clare-gerada-final-keynote-
    speech.aspx

40 http://www.rcgp.org.uk/campaign-home.aspx .

41 http://www.theguardian.com/society/2014/mar/23/family-doctor-service-
    brink-extinction.

42 http://www.rcgp.org.uk/news/2014/april/funding-for-general-practice-
    set-to-plummet-by-fifth-by-2017.aspx.

43 http://press.conservatives.com/post/98811391555/jeremy-hunt-speech-
    to-conservative-party-conference.

44 http://www.pulsetoday.co.uk/home/finance-and-practice-life-news/tens-
    of-thousands-of-gps-on-brink-of-early-retirement-bma-finds/20006182.
    article#.VFJdNYfCSnh.

45 http://www.theguardian.com/society/2014/mar/24/family-doctors-
    considering-early-retirement.

46 http://www.pulsetoday.co.uk/home/finance-and-practice-life-news/tens-
    of-thousands-of-gps-on-brink-of-early-retirement-bma-finds/20006182.

article#.VFJjHIfCSng.

47 http://careers.bmj.com/careers/advice/view-article.html?id=20018342.

48 http://www.pulsetoday.co.uk/your-practice/practice-topics/education/
    health-secretary-announces-independent-review-to-assess-gaps-in-gp-
    workforce/20008103.article#.VFJgc4fCSng.

49 http://bma.org.uk/news-views-analysis/news/2014/october/government-
    seeks-answers-on-gp-shortage.

50 http://www.pulsetoday.co.uk/home/stop-practice-closures/one-in-
    20-gps-considering-closing-their-practice-by-next-spring/20008370.
    article?msgid=38019#.VHM1KI1ybxk.

Chapter 5

1   http://www.wired-gov.net/wg/wg-news-1.nsf/0/033E9E6D28D4372F802579
    0300307B6B?OpenDocument.

2   http://www.theguardian.com/society/2014/jul/26/nhs-managers-
    redundancy-payments-total?CMP=twt_gu.

3   http://news.bbc.co.uk/1/hi/health/8290861.stm.

4   http://www.theguardian.com/politics/2010/jul/11/andrew-lansley-jobs-
    purge-nhs.

5   http://blogs.channel4.com/factcheck/factcheck-the-truth-about-the-nhs-
    reform-bill-myths/8160.

6   http://www.kingsfund.org.uk/current-projects/leadership-commission/
    the-changing-role-of

7   http://www.gponline.com/rcgp-urges-doh-slow-down-health-bill/
    article/1078261.

8   http://www.theguardian.com/society/2014/jul/26/nhs-managers-
    redundancy-payments-total?CMP=twt_gu.

9   https://fullfact.org/factchecks/andrew_lansley_and_the_cost_of_nhs_
    bureaucracy-1570.

10 http://www.nhsforsale.info/database/impact-database/increased-
    bureaucracy.html.

11 https://www.opendemocracy.net/ournhs/gary-walker/kings-fund-
    suggests-nhs-fees-but-is-it-really-independent..

12 https://www.gov.uk/government/...data/.../DH-6083-PCCR-IA-Final.pdf.

13 http://nhsrationing.org/tag/competitive-tendering/.

14 http://www.theguardian.com/healthcare-network/2014/feb/26/nhs-
    competitive-tendering-process.

15 http://andyburnhammp.blogspot.co.uk/2013/12/nhs-check-spiralling-
    cost-of-camerons.html.

16 Ibid.

17 http://www.telegraph.co.uk/news/politics/11282888/NHS-spending-on-management-consultants-doubles-under-Coalition.html.

18 www.bmj.com/content/349/bmj.g7243.

19 http://www.pharmafile.com/news/174130/nhs-must-tackle-tsunami-bureaucracy.

20 http://www.theguardian.com/healthcare-network/2013/mar/25/how-bureaucracy-nhs-reduced.

21 http://www.telegraph.co.uk/health/healthnews/10462858/NHS-doctors-spend-10-hours-a-week-on-bureaucracy.html; http://www.bbc.co.uk/news/health-22206882.

Chapter 6

1   17 January 2011, http://www.channel4.com/news/the-nhs-reforms-and-you.

2   8 June 2011; www.hospitaldr.co.uk/features/lansley-interview-we-shouldnt-separate-care-and-management.

3   Conservativehome. 25 April 2009: 'Lansley promises to secure spending on healthcare as part of a ten point SAVE OUR NHS plan', http://conservativehome.blogs.com/torydiary/healthcare/.

4   Lansley, A. 2010. Speech to NHS Confederation conference 24 June 2010, *Health Policy Insight*, http://www.healthpolicyinsight.com/?q=node/583.

5   People's Inquiry into London's NHS 2014. *London's NHS at the Crossroads*, http://www.peoplesinquiry.org/pdf/NHSattheCrossroadsfulldoc.pdf, p. 39 .

6   Leys C. Player, S. 2008. *Confuse and Conceal: the NHS and Independent Sector Treatment Centres*, Merlin Press, London.

7   Leys, C., Player S. 2011. *The Plot Against the NHS,* Merlin Press, London.

8   https://www.gov.uk/government/publications/statutory-guidance-for-trust-special-administrators-appointed-to-nhs-trusts.

9   Fisher B. 2013. 'Clause 118 of care bill threatens hospitals with downsizing or closure', *Guardian,* 18 December, http://www.theguardian.com/healthcare-network/2013/dec/18/care-bill-clause-118-threatens-hospitals.

10 For some historical background see Lister J. 2008. *The NHS after 60, For patients or profits?* Middlesex University Press.

11 Rathfelder M. 2013. *Patient voice?* Socialist Health Association, 6 April, http://www.sochealth.co.uk/2013/04/06/patient-voice/.

12 Lister J. 1998. *Casting Care Aside*, A response to Worcestershire Health Authority's proposals for rationalisation of hospital services, researched

for Wyre Forest District Council, http://www.healthemergency.org.uk/
pdf/WORCS%20Kidderminster.pdf.

13 Lister J. 2003. *Journalists Briefing Pack: What's the argument
over Foundation Trusts?* London Health Emergency, http://www.
healthemergency.org.uk/pdf/journospackandfreedoms.pdf.

14 Lister J. 2009a. *Healthworkers Guide to World Class Commissioning*,
UNISON Eastern Region, http://www.healthemergency.org.uk/
workingwu/Healthworkersguide.pdf; Lister J. 2009b. *What are they
doing to our NHS?* Public Information Sheet, UNISON Eastern Region,
http://www.healthemergency.org.uk/workingwu/Publicguide.pdf; Lister
J. 2008. *Fragmenting the NHS, Dangers to staff, services and patients
from 'social enterprises'*, UNISON Oxfordshire Health Branch, http://
www.healthemergency.org.uk/workingwu/SocialEnterprisepamphlet.
pdf.

15 Lister J. 2009c. UNISON *Eastern Eye*, UNISON Eastern Region, http://
www.healthemergency.org.uk/workingwu/TCS4pager.pdf.

16 Department of Health Social Enterprise Unit. 2008. *Social Enterprise
– Making a Difference*, http://www.socialenterprise.org.uk/uploads/
files/2011/11/social_enteprise_making_a_difference_guide.pdf.

17 Burnham A. 2009. Speech by the Rt Hon Andy Burnham, Secretary
of State for Health, 17 September 2009 to the King's Fund, http://
webarchive.nationalarchives.gov.uk/+/www.dh.gov.uk/en/MediaCentre/
Speeches/DH_105366.

18 *Health Emergency*, 2008. No. 65, Summer, http://www.healthemergency.
org.uk/he-issues/he65.pdf; Lister J. 2007. *Under the Knife, a response
to the A Picture of Health review*, http://www.healthemergency.org.uk/
workingwu/Undertheknife.pdf.

19 *Nursing in Practice*, 2008. 'Lord Darzi sets out tough rules for changes in
the NHS', 9 May, http://www.nursinginpractice.com/article/lord-darzi-
sets-out-tough-rules-changes-nhs.

20 http://www.kingsfund.org.uk/sites/files/kf/dealing-with-financially-
unsustainable-providers-anna-dixon-tony-harrison-sept12.pdf.

21 Trust Special Administrator, 2013. *Securing sustainable NHS services:
the Trust Special Administrator's report on South London Healthcare
NHS Trust and the NHS in south east London*, http://moderngov.
southwark.gov.uk/documents/s35012/TSA%20Final%20Report.pdf.

22 http://www.leighday.co.uk/News/2013/July-2013/High-Court-quashes-
decision-by-Jeremy-Hunt-to-clos.

23 BBC News, 2014. MPs grant powers to close local hospitals 11 March,
http://www.bbc.co.uk/news/health-26531807.

24 Standfield C. 2013. Written evidence to the People's Inquiry

into London's NHS, http://www.peoplesinquiry.org/pdf/PE-ColinStandfielddossier.pdf.

25 BBC News, 2013. Ealing Council votes for A&E closures plan referral, 6 March, http://www.bbc.co.uk/news/uk-england-london-21664279.

26 Lydall R. 2013. 'Two London hospital A&E units axed while two more could have their services cut', *Evening Standard* October 30, http://www.standard.co.uk/news/health/two-london-hospital-ae-units-axed-while-two-more-could-have-their-services-cut-8913230.html.

27 Independent Reconfiguration Panel, 2013. *Advice on Shaping A Healthier Future proposals for changes to NHS services in North West London* http://healthwatchhillingdon.org.uk/wp-content/uploads/downloads/2013/10/SaHF_IRP_advice_Report_13.09.13.pdf.

28 Adams, S. 2014. 'A&E unit in London faces axe ... after PM promised personally it would stay open', *Daily Mail*, 7 September, http://www.dailymail.co.uk/news/article-2746480/A-E-unit-London-faces-axe-PM-promised-personally-stay-open.html.

29 http://www.andyslaughter.co.uk/devastating_news_for_local_health_service_as_a_e_closures_and_charing_cross_demolition_get_go_ahead.

30 http://www.gponline.com/gp-poll-halts-hospital-reconfiguration/article/1222046.

31 https://www.gov.uk/government/uploads/system/uploads/attachment_data/file/356383/BM1492_NHSFT_quarterly_performance.pdf.

32 Lister J. 2014b. *London's NHS at the Crossroads: the report of the Peoples Inquiry into London's NHS. Unite London & Eastern Region*. Full report: http://www.peoplesinquiry.org/pdf/NHSattheCrossroadsfulldoc.pdf.

Chapter 7

1 https://www.gov.uk/government/news/a-more-transparent-and-safer-nhs-for-patients.

2 https://www.gov.uk/government/uploads/system/uploads/attachment_data/file/213823/dh_117794.pdf.

3 Department of Health. 2010. Andrew Lansley announces NHS management costs to be slashed, Press release, copy available http://www.lmc.org.uk/article.php?group_id=1849.

4 Available http://www.healthpolicyinsight.com/?q=node.

5 For one vivid example see Lister J, 2013. Dead Weight: Mid Yorkshire Hospital Trust's impossible £2bn PFI burden, Mid Yorkshire Hospitals Branch of UNISON, available http://www.healthemergency.org.uk/pdf/DeadWeight.pdf.

6   BBC News, 15 May 2012, NHS risk register veto 'unjustified', http://www.
     bbc.co.uk/news/health-18071681.

7   Department of Health. 8 May 2012. Risk register will not be published,
     Press Release, available https://www.gov.uk/government/news/risk-
     register-will-not-be-published.

8   Department of Health. May 2012. Transition Programme Risks: Review
     of November 2010 risk register, https://www.gov.uk/government/
     uploads/system/uploads/attachment_data/file/216553/dh_133980.pdf.

9   http://origin.library.constantcontact.com/download/get/
     file/1102665899193-1592/Health-Bill-Transition-Risk-Register-NC-15-Oct-
     10-Dept-Bd-Version-v1.pdf.

10   Gainsbury S. 2009. NHS spending: 'McKinsey exposes hard choices to
     save £20bn', *Health Service Journal* 10 September, http://www.hsj.co.uk/
     news/policy/nhs-spending-mckinsey-exposes-hard-choices-to-save-
     20bn/5005952.article#.

11   Stevens S. October 2014. 'Five Year Forward View', NHS England, http://
     www.england.nhs.uk/wp-content/uploads/2014/10/5yfv-web.pdf.

12   http://www.healthemergency.org.uk/pdf/McKinsey%20affordability%20
     document%20for%20NHS%20London%202009.pdf.

13   http://www.nhsconfed.org/news/2014/03/hold-your-ground-for-a-
     settlement-that-meets-the-nhs-mandate-mental-health-leaders-urged.

14   https://www.gov.uk/government/uploads/system/uploads/attachment_
     data/file/281250/Closing_the_gap_V2_-_17_Feb_2014.pdf.

15   Clark E. 2014. 'GP service under 'severe threat of extinction', says top
     doctor', *The Independent*, 23 March, available http://www.independent.
     co.uk/news/uk/home-news/gp-service-under-severe-threat-of-
     extinction-says-top-doctor-9210654.html.

16   Lind S. 2014. 'East London campaign to save GP practices expands with
     new rally', *Pulse*, 27 June, available http://www.pulsetoday.co.uk/home/
     finance-and-practice-life-news/east-london-campaign-to-save-gp-
     practices-expands-with-new-rally/20007124.article#.VFzpt41ybxk.

17   http://www.england.nhs.uk/london/wp-content/uploads/sites/8/2013/11/
     Call-Action-ACCESSIBLE.pdf.

18   http://www.rcgp.org.uk/news/2014/october/over-500-surgeries-at-risk-of-
     closure-as-gp-workforce-crisis-deepens.aspx.

19   The issue is discussed in the full report of the People's Inquiry into
     London's NHS (March 2014) available http://www.peoplesinquiry.org/
     pdf/NHSattheCrossroadsfulldoc.pdf.

20   Large, Z. July 2014. 'Major failings' in CAMHS Tier Four services, a new
     review reveals, Young Minds, http://www.youngminds.org.uk/news/
     blog/2137_major_failings_in_camhs_tier_four_services_a_new_review_

reveals.

21 Lind S. 2014. 'NHS England to drop "cash for dementia diagnoses scheme', *Pulse* 26 November http://www.pulsetoday.co.uk/home/finance-and-practice-life-news/nhs-england-to-drop-cash-for-dementia-diagnoses-scheme/20008567.article#.VHYgKo1ybxk.

22 National Audit Office. November 2014. The financial sustainability of NHS bodies. http://www.nao.org.uk/report/financial-sustainability-nhs-bodies-2/.

23 Roderick, P, Pollock, AM. 2014. 'A wolf in sheep's clothing: how Monitor is using licensing powers to reduce hospital and community service in England under the guise of continuity', *BMJ* 7 October, doi: 10.1136/bmj.g5603.

24 Committee of Public Accounts. 2014. Monitor, regulating NHS Foundation Trusts, The Stationery Office, July 4, available http://www.parliament.uk/business/committees/committees-a-z/commons-select/public-accounts-committee/news/monitor-regulating-nhs-foundation-trusts-report/.

25 http://www.networks.nhs.uk/nhs-networks/ahp-networks/documents/AQP%20guidance.pdf/view.

26 http://www.england.nhs.uk/wp-content/uploads/2013/11/aqp-sup-com-serv.pdf.

27 https://www.nhs.uk/Services/Trusts/Overview/DefaultView.aspx?id=3240 accessed 26/11/14.

28 Syal, R., Bowers, S., Wintour, P., and Jones, S. 2013. 'Margaret Hodge urges accountancy code of practice over role in tax laws theguardian.com', *The Guardian*, April 26, http://www.theguardian.com/business/2013/apr/26/margaret-hodge-accountancy-code-practice.

29 https://www.gov.uk/government/organisations/monitor/about/our-governance.

30 Lilley R. 2014. No one answers, nhsmanagers.net, 12 August, http://archive.constantcontact.com/fs136/1102665899193/archive/1118177786207.html.

31 Borland S. 2014. 'NHS watchdog chief goes private for hip Operation', *Daily Mail*, April 19, available http://www.dailymail.co.uk/...8139/NHS-watchdog-chief-goes-private-hip-operation-avoiding-three-month-wait-patients-face-hospitals-hes-meant-improving.html.

32 Hazell W. 2014. CQC chair: 30 acutes could end up in special measures, *Health Service Journal* March 14, available £ http://www.hsj.co.uk/news/cqc-chair-30-acutes-could-end-up-in-special-measures/5068936.article#.VFz7TY1ybxk.

33 Commons Health Committee. 2012. http://www.publications.parliament.

uk/pa/cm201012/cmselect/cmhealth/1816/181608.htm#note82 ; The
Lancet, 18 January 2012, *Offline: The scandal of device regulation in the
UK.*

34 Monbiot G. 2013. This transatlantic trade deal is a full-frontal assault
on democracy, *The Guardian*, November 4, http://www.theguardian.
com/commentisfree/2013/nov/04/us-trade-deal-full-frontal-assault-on-
democracy.

35 http://www.huffingtonpost.co.uk/2014/07/03/ttip-eu-us-trade-deal-unite-
union_n_5554227.html.

36 Barnes S. 2014.'Patient transport service fails to improv'e, *HSJ*, 25
July, available (£) http://www.hsj.co.uk/hsj-local/ccgs/nhs-west-
kent-ccg/patient-transport-service-fails-to-improve/5073302.article#.
VHYWhl1ybxk.

Chapter 8

1   11 May 2011, http://www.telegraph.co.uk/news/politics/8506816/Why-
the-NHS-needs-competition.html.

2   Letwin O. 1988. *Privatising the World. A Study of International
Privatisation in Theory and Practice*, London: Cassell, p. 34.

3   21 November 1864, letter to Col. William F. Elkins.

4   1 September 2014, http://www.marlboroughnewsonline.co.uk/features/
health-nhs/3391-the-nhs-and-privatisation-now-gp-practices-will-be-
opened-up-to-private-providers.

5   Pollock, Allyson M. 2005. *NHS Plc: The Privatisation of Our Health Care*,
London: Verso; and Leys, Colin & Player, Stewart. 2011. *The Plot against
the NHS*, London: Merlin Press.

6   Woolhandler & Himmelstein. 2007. *British Medical Journal*,
2007;335:1126.

7   www.bjj.boneandjoint.org.uk/content/91-B/9/1154.abstract.

8   http://www.hospitaldr.co.uk/features/istc-programme-at-a-cross-roads-
over-damning-evidence.

9   http://www.bbc.co.uk/news/uk-england-beds-bucks-herts-24106914;
and http://www.theguardian.com/society/2012/oct/28/nhs-deaths-clinic-
carillion.

10 Ibid.

11 http://www.theguardian.com/society/2012/aug/12/nhs-private-carillion-
sight-clinicenta?guni=Article:in%20body%20link.

12 Ibid.

13 Ibid.

14 http://www.thebureauinvestigates.com/2014/06/02/appalling-service-

provided-by-healthcare-at-home-leaves-patients-without-drugs/.

15 chpi.org.uk/patientsafety/.

16 BMJ2014;349:g5241.

17 http://www.theguardian.com/society/2014/aug/14/nhs-eye-operations-private-provider-musgrove.

18 http://www.theguardian.com/society/2014/oct/15/hospital-refuses-publish-report-outsourced-eye-operation-problems.

19 http://www.theguardian.com/uk-news/2014/oct/17/musgrove-park-hospital-eye-surgeries-taunton-somerset; http://www.theguardian.com/society/2014/oct/16/leaked-report-cataract-surgery-revealed.

20 BMJ2014;348:g4184.

21 http://www.economist.com/news/united-states/21603078-why-thieves-love-americas-health-care-system-272-billion-swindle.

22 http://www.bmj.com/press-releases/2013/03/12/bmj-investigation-finds-gp-conflicts-interest-"rife"-commissioning-boards.

23 http://www.pulsetoday.co.uk/commissioning/commissioning-topics/ccgs/revealed-one-in-five-gps-on-ccg-boards-has-financial-interest-in-a-current-provider/20004369.article.

24 http://www.theargus.co.uk/news/11508955.Privatised_NHS_service_decision_is_under_review/.

25 http://www.healthinvestor.co.uk/ShowArticle.aspx?ID=3617.

26 http://articles.baltimoresun.com/2011-02-08/health/bs-bz-hancock-orthopod-mris-20110208_1_ct-mri-scans-maryland-law; http://www.managedcaremag.com/content/enduring-temptation-physician-self-referral.

27 http://www.fbi.gov/about-us/investigate/white_collar/health-care-fraud.

28 BMJ2009;338:b1421; the House of Commons Health Committee had concluded that lack of data made an assessment of the programme impossible, and in July 2007 the Healthcare Commission could not report on quality of care because English ISTCs failed to return and comply with Hospital Episode Statistics data requirements. Pollock and Kirkwood based their conclusions on information obtained in Scotland. For more information about the ISTC programme see Leys, Colin & Player, Stewart. 2008. *Confuse and Conceal*, London: Merlin Press.

29 http://www.nhsforsale.info/database/impact-database/less-fair/cherry-picking.html; http://www.thebureauinvestigates.com/2011/06/14/5899/.

30 http://www.ft.com/cms/s/fec81b5c-0bef-11e2-8e06-00144feabdc0,Authorised=false.html?_i_location=http%3A%2F%2Fwww.ft.com%2Fcms%2Fs%2F0%2Ffec81b5c-0bef-11e2-8e06-00144feabdc0.html%3Fsiteedition%3Duk&siteedition=uk&_i_referer=http%3A%2F%2Fwww.nhsforsale.info%2Fdatabase%2Fimpact-

database%2Fless-fair%2Fcherry-picking.html#axzz2l5rooPsl.
31 http://www.nhsforsale.info/database/impact-database/less-fair/cherry-picking.html.
32 https://sites.google.com/site/nhsfuture/Home/debunking-the-myths/myth-10.
33 http://www.telegraph.co.uk/health/nhs/11053982/Superior-private-health-is-a-myth.html#disqus_thread
34 http://www.telegraph.co.uk/news/politics/labour/6611887/The-doctor-who-died-as-a-result-of-Labours-ISTCs.html.
35 http://www.theguardian.com/world/2012/feb/24/breast-implant-scandal-patients-nhs.
36 http://www.theguardian.com/uk/2012/nov/28/cosmetic-surgery-millionaire-offshore-firm.
37 http://www.dailymail.co.uk/news/article-2234621/Faulty-breast-implant-firm-plunges-bankruptcy--avoid-paying-millions-1-700-victims.html.
38 Ibid.
39 http://www.telegraph.co.uk/health/healthnews/9334459/Breast-implant-scandal-has-cost-taxpayer-3m.html.
40 http://www.pulsetoday.co.uk/gps-lose-out-on-apms-contracts-despite-scoring-higher-than-private-firms/10970653.article#.VD4T6mIayK0.
41 http://www.theguardian.com/society/2012/dec/19/when-privitisation-gp-practices-wrong.
42 Ibid.
43 Ibid.
44 http://www.camdennewjournal.com/news/2012/feb/gp-surgery-was-sold-us-health-company-set-close.
45 http://www.nhsforsale.info/private-providers/private-provider-profiles-2/the-practice-plc.html.
46 http://www.chroniclelive.co.uk/news/north-east-news/private-company-exiting-newcastle-gp-7067521.
47 http://www.kentonline.co.uk/thanet/news/threat-to-surgery-20444/.
48 http://www.thanetgazette.co.uk/Concordia-Health-pull-contract-Broadway-Practice/story-21657524-detail/story.html; http://www.dover-express.co.uk/GP-s-fury-medical-chaos/story-24278761-detail/story.html.
49 BMJ2014;349:g5248.
50 http://www.thebureauinvestigates.com/2012/09/04/nhs-pfi-firms-avoid-millions-in-tax/.
51 Ibid.
52 http://www.independent.co.uk/news/uk/home-news/tax-special-investigation-firms-running-nhs-care-services-avoiding-millions-in-tax-8892925.html.

53 http://www.independent.co.uk/news/uk/politics/exclusive-how-private-firms-make-quick-killing-from-pfi-9488351.html.

54 Ibid.

55 https://www.opendemocracy.net/ourkingdom/margaret-hodge/parliamentary-watchdog-too-often-private-sector-contractors%27-ethical-stand.

56 See 'The end of medicine as a profession?' in Raymond Tallis: *Hippocratic Oaths. Medicine and its Discontents* London: Atlantic, 2004.

57 http://www.mirror.co.uk/lifestyle/health/bupa-harming-nhs-offering-patients-3390254#ixzz2yribYvpu.

58 http://www.bmj.com/content/347/bmj.f5933.

59 http://www.bmj.com/content/346/bmj.f1501.

60 http://www.theguardian.com/business/2013/jul/29/serco-biggest-company-never-heard-of.

61 http://www.nhsforsale.info/private-providers/private-provider-profiles-2/serco.html.

62 http://www.theguardian.com/business/2013/jul/29/serco-biggest-company-never-heard-of.

63 http://www.parliament.uk/business/committees/committees-a-z/commons-select/public-accounts-committee/news/out-of-hours-gp-service-in-cornwall/.

64 Ibid; see also http://www.theguardian.com/society/2012/may/25/serco-investigated-claims-unsafe-hours-gp and http://www.theguardian.com/society/2012/sep/20/serco-nhs-false-data-gps.

65 Ibid.

66 http://www.ft.com/fastft/81542/post-81542.

67 http://www.bmj.com/content/348/bmj.g1167.

68 http://www.hsj.co.uk/news/serco-seeks-nhs-help-to-fill-vacancies/5065381.article.

69 http://www.bmj.com/content/348/bmj.g1167.

70 http://www.leftfootforward.org/2014/05/public-want-serco-banned-from-government-

71 http://www.healthinvestor.co.uk/ShowArticle.aspx?ID=3501.

72 http://www.theguardian.com/public-leaders-network/2014/apr/10/serco-employees-targets-treated-children-contracts.

73 http://www.theguardian.com/business/2013/jul/29/serco-biggest-company-never-heard-of.

74 http://www.ft.com/intl/cms/s/0/69c31024-4af1-11e3-8c4c-00144feabdc0.html.

75 http://www.independent.co.uk/news/uk/politics/nhs-services-cut-in-nottingham-after-doctors-quit-rather-than-work-for-private-

firm-9931763.html.

76   Ibid.

77   http://www.ft.com/intl/cms/s/0/69c31024-4af1-11e3-8c4c-00144feabdc0.
     html.

Chapter 9

1   BBC, Andrew Lansley when confronted by a protester, 20 February 2012,
    http://www.bbc.co.uk/news/uk-17093082.

2   10 September 2014,; http://www.independent.co.uk/news/uk/
    politics/hospital-emergency-departments-hunt-has-sympathy-for-
    charging-drunks-9725164.html; http://www.dailymail.co.uk/health/
    article-2751754/Charge-drunks-end-A-E-Jeremy-Hunt-says-taxpayers-
    not-foot-bill-people-gone-night-out.html; https://www.youtube.com/
    watch?v=Y96OrC4kCc8.

3   June 2011, http://www.libdems.org.uk/nick_clegg_speech_how_we_re_
    protecting_our_nhs. http://www.libdemvoice.org/nick-cleggs-speech-
    on-nhs-reforms-weve-listened-weve-learned-24447.html

4   Bevan, Aneurin. 1952. *In place of fear*, London, Heinemann.

5   http://www.ipsos-mori.com/researchpublications/researcharchive/2939/
    Britons-are-more-proud-of-their-history-NHS-and-army-than-the-Royal-
    Family.aspx.

6   http://www.nextleft.org/2011/04/nhs-makes-socialists-of-us-all-says.html.

7   http://www.theepochtimes.com/n2/united-kingdom/cameron-defends-
    whole-scale-nhs-reform-49611.html; http://new.muslimnews.co.uk/
    newspaper/home-news/exclusive-interview-hunt-denies-support-for-
    denationalisation-of-nhs/.

8   http://www.pulsetoday.co.uk/political/political-news/department-of-
    health-denies-nhs-privatisation-claims/20007389.article#.VB3dR_ldWHk.

9   http://www.bbc.com/news/uk-england-manchester-24286582; http://
    www.bbc.com/news/uk-england-29094093.

10 http://liberalconspiracy.org/2011/06/03/worried-john-redwood-disowns-
    his-own-nhs-pamphlet/.

11 Finkelstein, Daniel. 14 April 2010. 'The wizard behind Cameron's little
    blue book'. *The Times* (London); 'Profiles of men trying to negotiate a
    Tory-Lib Dem deal'. BBC News (London). 10 May 2010.

12 http://www.independent.co.uk/life-style/health-and-families/health-
    news/letwin-nhs-will-not-exist-under-tories-6168295.html.

13 Jeremy Hunt is also rumoured to have objected to Danny Boyle's
    Opening Ceremony for the Olympic Games, in which hundreds
    of dancing Great Ormond Street nurses celebrated the post-war

creation of the NHS. Hunt is reported to have tried to persuade
the director to remove the sections featuring the NHS. http://www.
thebureauinvestigates.com/2012/09/11/opinion-the-new-health-
secretary-and-the-650m-private-healthcare-takeover/.

14   http://www.theguardian.com/commentisfree/2012/sep/06/jeremy-hunt-
in-tray-wipe-smile or http://www.gponline.com/gps-need-know-health-
secretary-jeremy-hunt/article/1148534.

15   https://yougov.co.uk/news/2013/11/04/nationalise-energy-and-rail-
companies-say-public/.

16   For a collection of peers' and MPs' quotes in support of the HSC Act
listed alongside their interests in the private heath industry http://
socialinvestigations.blogspot.co.uk/p/lords-and-mps-quotes-on-health-
and.html

17   http://www.bmj.com/content/342/bmj.d2996?sso=.

18   Muschell. J. 1995. Technical Briefing Note on Privatization in Health,
WHO/TFHE/TBN/95.1.

19   BMJ2013;346:f1322.

20   BMJ2013;346:f1608.

21   http://www.pulsetoday.co.uk/commissioning/85-of-gps-believe-nhs-will-
be-privatised-within-ten-years/20007870.article#.VI71z_msWHk.

22   http://www.peoplesnhs.org/.

23   http://www.nhsforsale.info/privatisation-list.html.

24   BMJ2013;347:f4476.

25   http://www.bbc.co.uk/news/health-25660555.

26   http://www.unitetheunion.org/news/explosion-in-nhs-sell-off-just-one-
year-on-from-governments-changes/

27   BMJ2014;349:g7606

28   Personal communication from John Lister.

29   Personal communication.

30   m.huffpost.com/uk/entry/5866352.

31   http://www.theguardian.com/business/2013/jul/18/bain-capital-plasma-
resources-uk.

32   *Association of Clinical Pathologists News* Summer 2013, http://www.
pathologists.org.uk/publications.aspx?id=129.

33   http://www.parliament.uk/edm/2012-13/1164.

34   Ibid.

35   http://www.theguardian.com/society/2013/dec/29/cable-hunt-nhs-
privatised-plasma.

36   *Association of Clinical Pathologists News*, Summer 2013 http://www.
pathologists.org.uk/publications.aspx?id=129.

37   http://www.theguardian.com/commentisfree/2014/feb/08/britain-private-

sector-public-sector-ethics-customers.

38 http://webarchive.nationalarchives.gov.uk/+/www.dh.gov.uk/ab/Archive/IRNHSPS/index.htm.

39 http://www.theguardian.com/society/2012/sep/30/pathology-labs-takeover-failures#.

40 http://www.corporatewatch.org.uk/?q=node/4105%3f

41 http://www.independent.co.uk/news/uk/politics/exclusive-overcharging-by-outsourcing-giant-serco-costs-nhs-millions-9695342.html.

42 http://www.gponline.com/exclusive-private-firms-will-run-10-gp-practices-2014/article/1093504.

43 http://www.ft.com/cms/s/0/657b30e6-357a-11e3-952b-00144feab7de.html?siteedition=uk#ixzz3MAoIgODZ.

44 http://www.unison.org.uk/news/unison-fights-the-privatisation-of-primary-care-support-services.

45 http://www.thebureauinvestigates.com/2012/09/11/opinion-the-new-health-secretary-and-the-650m-private-healthcare-takeover/; BMJ2012;344:e2605.

46 BMJ2014;349:g4640.

47 http://www.huntspost.co.uk/news/staff_survey_of_hinchingbrooke_hospital_highlights_employees_concerns_1_3403534.

48 http://www.nao.org.uk/report/the-franchising-of-hinchingbrooke-health-care-nhs-trust/; http://www.hsj.co.uk/news/finance/exclusive-nhs-trust-under-private-management-faces-deficit-again/5069465.article#.U0sNClego8Y.

49 http://www.cambridge-news.co.uk/Car-park-Hinchingbrooke-Hospital-sold-housing-development/story-22821451-detail/story.html.

50 https://www.opendemocracy.net/ournhs/richard-grimes/why-is-government-preparing-for-dramatic-rise-in-nhs-patients-going-private; http://www.bbc.co.uk/news/health-16337904.

51 http://www.foundationtrustnetwork.org/news/enterprise-in-the-nhs-given-a-freer-rein/.

52 https://www.opendemocracy.net/ournhs/richard-grimes/why-is-government-preparing-for-dramatic-rise-in-nhs-patients-going-private.

53 http://www.theguardian.com/society/2014/sep/19/nhs-hospitals-waiting-time-demand-monitor.

54 http://www.theguardian.com/society/2014/apr/16/britain-fewer-hospital-beds-european-oecd; http://www.theguardian.com/society/2014/may/13/cuts-hospital-beds-nhs-false-economy-community-based-services.

55 BMJ2014;348:g2777.

56 http://www.theguardian.com/commentisfree/2012/aug/21/nhs-brand-private-profits.

57 http://www.theguardian.com/society/2014/jan/21/nhs-private-firms-may-help-hospital-patient-surge.
58 Ibid.
59 http://www.dailymail.co.uk/news/article-2549920/Struggling-NHS-hospitals-face-330m-red-44-cent-predict-debt-end-month.html.
60 BMJ2012;345:e7510.
61 BMJ2014;349:g5150.
62 http://www.thirdsector.co.uk/francis-maude-unveils-details-10m-mutuals-programme/policy-and-politics/article/1107775.
63 http://www.bmj.com/content/347/bmj.f4524.
64 Ibid.
65 Ibid.
66 BMJ2014;348:g2706.
67 https://www.betterasone.co.uk.
68 BMJ2012;344:e2605.
69 http://saveourpublicservices.co.uk/virgin-keep-out.php; http://www.brixtonbuzz.com/2013/11/brixton-protest-against-virgins-takeover-of-nhs-healthcare-services-photos-from-saturdays-flashmob/; http://www.youtube.com/watch?v=0zQ-2evkKzI.
70 http://www.bbc.co.uk/news/uk-england-cambridgeshire-23948457.
71 http://www.gmb.org.uk/newsroom/nhs-is-preferred-bidder-in-cambridgeshire; http://www.bbc.co.uk/news/uk-england-cambridgeshire-29439924.
72 http://www.theguardian.com/uk-news/2014/jul/02/cancer-care-nhs-outsourcing-ccgs-unison-virgin.
73 https://www.opendemocracy.net/ournhs/clive-peedell/outsourcing-cancer-care-biggest-and-most-reckless-nhs-privatisation-yet.
74 Ibid.
75 http://www.chichester.co.uk/news/local/update-235m-orthopaedic-contract-awarded-to-bupa-1-6279559#.VAjXXVUzIk9.twitter.
76 http://www.bognor.co.uk/news/local/a-e-sos-bupa-csh-contract-a-bad-decision-for-patients-1-6334245#.VC5BPSV-6Rw.twitter.
77 http://www.coastalwestsussexccg.nhs.uk/domains/coastal-west-sussex-ccg.org.uk/local/media/images/medium/20140826_Declaration_of_Interest_Register_1.pdf.
78 http://www.nuffieldtrust.org.uk/summit/2009/speakers/patrick-carter.
79 http://www.dailymail.co.uk/news/article-2109907/NHS-fairness-tsar-urged-quit-doctors-conflict-following-799-000-payment-U-S-private-health-giant.html.
80 http://www.bbc.co.uk/news/health-26175151.
81 http://4bitnews.com/shh-bits/hypocrisy-sir-stuart-rose-nhs/?utm_

content=bufferdebab&utm_medium=social&utm_source=twitter. com&utm_campaign=buffer.

82 http://www.nhsforsale.info/database/impact-database/conflict-of-interest/Monitor.html.

83 http://www.telegraph.co.uk/news/politics/conservative/11264425/ Stephen-Dorrell-MP-faces-calls-to-resign-over-conflict-of-interest.html.

84 http://www.mirror.co.uk/news/uk-news/david-cameron-stepped-up-plans-2073843.

85 BMJ2012;344:e2905.

86 https://twitter.com/h_jarman/status/428198335883669505/photo/1

87 BMJ2012;344:e2905; http://www.dailymail.co.uk/news/article-2099940/ NHS-health-reforms-Extent-McKinsey--Companys-role-Andrew-Lansleys-proposals.html.

88 http://www.theguardian.com/uk-news/the-northerner/2014/apr/23/999-call--recreate-jarrow-march-to-protest-at-nhs-privatisation?CMP=twt_gu.

89 http://yougov.co.uk/news/2013/11/04/nationalise-energy-and-rail-companies-say-public/.

90 http://www.standard.co.uk/news/health/80-per-cent-of-voters-would-pay-more-to-save-the-nhs-from-privatisation-9760941.html.

91 http://www.theguardian.com/commentisfree/2014/feb/08/britain-private-sector-public-sector-ethics-customers.

92 Relman AS. 2007. 'Medical professionalism in a commercialized health care market.' *JAMA* 2007;298:2688-70.

Chapter 10

1 http://www.dailymail.co.uk/news/article-1240061/Cameron-fires-starting-gun-election-launches-Tory-Year-Change-campaign.html.

2 *Bexley Times*, 'Possible services cash cut slammed', 25 February 2009: http://www.bexleytimes.co.uk/news/possible_services_cash_cut_slammed_1_609395.

3 Donnelly, L. 2014. 'Dozens of maternity and A&E units shut', *Daily Telegraph*, 26 October, http://www.telegraph.co.uk/journalists/laura-donnelly/11184764/Dozens-of-maternity-and-AandE-units-shut.html.

4 Figures from http://www.england.nhs.uk/statistics/statistical-work-areas/ bed-availability-and-occupancy/bed-data-overnight/.

5 *Commissioning Strategy Plan 2012 – 15*, Part A: Delivering Service Change in North West London, December 2011, http://www. northwestlondon.nhs.uk/_uploads/~filestore/665BD053-9434-490D-A085-29366356E0B6/3/%20NHS%20NWL%20Commissioning%20Strategy%20

Plan%20Part%20B.pdf.

6   Figures are taken from the *PreConsultation Business Case*,
      Volume 8, Appendix C, page 10 (20 June 2012): http://www.
      healthiernorthwestlondon.nhs.uk/sites/default/files/documents/PCBC-
      Vol08-AppC-v1.1.pdf .

7   *Commissioning Strategy Plan 2012 – 15*, Part B: The commissioning and
      provider landscape and NHS NWL's enabling plans NHS NW London,
      page 163, June 2012, http://goo.gl/6rCeL.

8   http://www.standard.co.uk/news/health/waiting-times-at-ae-at-west-
      london-hospitals-hit-a-record-after-closures-9850531.html.

9   Campbell D. 2012. 'NHS needs to close wards and hospitals to
      centralise care, says doctors' leader', *The Guardian*, July 24, http://www.
      theguardian.com/society/2012/jul/24/nhs-hospitals-need-to-close.

10   Smith, R. 2010. 'Do not downgrade A&Es: president of College of
      Emergency Medicine', *Daily Telegraph* 29 April, 2010, http://www.
      telegraph.co.uk/health/healthnews/7644567/Do-not-downgrade-AandEs-
      president-of-college-of-emergency-medicine.html,

11   http://www.healthemergency.org.uk/pdf/McKinsey%20affordability%20
      document%20for%20NHS%20London%202009.pdf.

12   Lister, J. 2014. *Briefing for Cynical Commissioning Groups*,
      Health Emergency, http://www.healthemergency.org.uk/pdf/
      CynicalCommissioningGroups1.pdf.

13   Healthcare for London, 2007. *A Framework for Action – Technical Paper*:
      http://www.healthemergency.org.uk/pdf/Technical%20report.pdf.

14   Healthcare for London, 2008. *Study of Unscheduled Care in 6 Primary
      Care Trusts Central Report*, http://www.healthemergency.org.uk/pdf/
      HfL-Study-of-Unscheduled-Care-in-6-PCTs-Central-Report.pdf.

15   *Primary Care and Emergency Departments*, http://www.
      healthemergency.org.uk/pdf/Primary%20Care%20and%20
      Emergency%20Departments.pdf.

16   Ibid, p. 4.

17   Ibid, p. 5.

18   Ibid, p. 8.

19   *Health Equalities Impact Assessment*, p. 24. https://www.gov.uk/
      government/uploads/system/uploads/attachment_data/file/213356/VOL-
      3-Appendix-L.pdf.

20   Lister, J. 2014. *Reasons to be Fearful*, a response to plans from
      Bedfordshire & Milton Keynes CCGs, UNISON Eastern Region, http://
      www.healthemergency.org.uk/pdf/1%20Bedfordshire4-pager%20
      August%202014.pdf.

21   *Integrated Strategic Plan 2010-2015, First Stage Report*, (Healthcare for

London), NHS London, January 2010, http://www.peoplesinquiry.org/
pdf/NHS%20London%20Integrated%20Strategic%20Plan%20smaller.
pdf. p.3.

22 http://www.hsj.co.uk/5046128.article?referrer=e2.
23 Lister, J. 2012. *NW London's NHS Under the Knife, a response to Shaping a Healthier Future*, http://www.healthemergency.org.uk/pdf/NorthWestLondonNHS-UndertheKnife.pdf.
24 http://www.healthiernorthwestlondon.nhs.uk/.
25 Lister, J. 2014. *Costly Savings, East Midlands Region UNISON*, http://www.healthemergency.org.uk/pdf/1%20Costly%20Savings%20updated%20final.pdf.
26 Lister, J. 2014. *Briefing for Cynical Commissioning Groups*, Health Emergency, http://www.healthemergency.org.uk/pdf/CynicalCommissioningGroups1.pdf.
27 The full 842 page report can be downloaded from: http://webarchive.nationalarchives.gov.uk/20130107105354/http:/www.dh.gov.uk/en/Publicationsandstatistics/Publications/PublicationsPolicyAndGuidance/DH_113018.
28 *Integrated Strategic Plan 2010-2015*, pp. 3-4.
29 Purdy, S. et al. 2012. *Interventions to reduce unplanned hospital admission: a series of systematic reviews: final report*. Bristol: University of Bristol, http://www.bristol.ac.uk/media-library/sites/primaryhealthcare/migrated/documents/unplannedadmissions.pdf.
30 Roland, M., Abel, G. 2012. *Reducing emergency admissions: are we on the right track?* BMJ 2012;345:e6017, 16 September, http://www.bmj.com/content/345/bmj.e6017.
31 Stevens, S. 2014. *Five Year Forward View*, NHS England, http://www.england.nhs.uk/wp-content/uploads/2014/10/5yfv-web.pdf.
32 http://www.nhshistory.com/Leading%20local%20change.pdf.

Chapter 11

1 http://www.bbc.co.uk/news/uk-politics-12250186.
2 http://www.independent.co.uk/life-style/health-and-families/health-news/letwin-nhs-will-not-exist-under-tories-6168295.html.
3 https://www.youtube.com/watch?v=nH2EmVGowCk.
4 https://www.ipsos-mori.com/Assets/Docs/Polls/Feb2013_Trust_Topline.PDF.
5 http://www.theguardian.com/society/2010/jul/12/nhs-private-companies-gps-funds.
6 http://socialinvestigations.blogspot.co.uk/.

7   http://socialinvestigations.blogspot.co.uk/2012/02/nhs-privatisation-
     compilation-of.html.
8   http://www.mirror.co.uk/news/uk-news/nhs-hospital-corporation-
     america-donates-2246513#.
9   http://www.peoplesnhs.org/lord-popat/.
10   http://www.theguardian.com/politics/2014/oct/03/healthcare-companies-
     links-tories-nhs-contracts.
11   http://www.theguardian.com/politics/2014/oct/03/healthcare-companies-
     links-tories-nhs-contracts.
12   http://www.telegraph.co.uk/news/newstopics/mps-expenses/6989408/
     Andrew-Lansley-bankrolled-by-private-healthcare-provider.html.
13   http://www.theguardian.com/education/2013/jan/10/gove-appoints-john-
     nash-education-minister; http://politicalscrapbook.net/2013/01/tory-
     donor-given-peerage-and-ministerial-job-john-nash-education.
14   http://www.parliament.uk/biographies/lords/lord-warner/1732.
15   http://www.theguardian.com/society/2013/apr/24/labour-peer-nhs-
     regulations.
16   http://tompride.co.uk/2013/04/23/why-lord-warner-really-supports-nhs-
     reform-hell-make-loads-of-money-from-it/.
17   It never ceases to amaze that politicians can make sweeping statements
     backed by little or no evidence and yet be allocated many column
     inches peddling their mischievous ideas without being challenged.
     Even the *Guardian* is not beyond criticism in this respect.
18   http://www.theguardian.com/commentisfree/2014/mar/31/10-pounds-
     each-save-nhs?INTCMP=ILCNETTXT3487.
19   Norman Warner, Jack O'Sullivan, 2014. *Solving the NHS care and cash
     crisis: Routes to health and care renewal*, London: Reform (available
     online).
20   http://www.itv.com/news/update/2014-03-31/labour-would-not-consider-
     nhs-monthly-charge.
21   http://www.bmj.com/content/321/7269/1101.1.
22   http://www.telegraph.co.uk/health/healthnews/9066483/Downing-Street-
     does-not-want-Andrew-Lansley-taken-out-and-shot.html.
23   http://www.telegraph.co.uk/news/10593106/Poverty-tsar-Alan-Milburn-
     makes-a-million.html.
24   http://www.accountancyage.com/aa/news/2270407/alan-milburn-takes-
     pwc-health-role.
25   http://www.lobbyingtransparency.org/15-blog/general/62-revolving-
     door-is-unhealthy.
26   http://www.theguardian.com/politics/2012/nov/23/david-cameron-
     privatisation-adviser-health-lobbyist.

27 Leys, Colin & Player, Stewart, 2011. *The Plot against the NHS*, London: Merlin, p. 15.

28 http://spendmatters.com/uk/exclusive-department-health-settle-court-ken-anderson-commercial-director/; http://www.dailymail.co.uk/news/article-1389609/NHS-troubleshooter-given-free-Porsche-exotic-holiday-sued-250-000.html.

29 http://www.theguardian.com/uk/2004/sep/30/politics.freedomofinformation.

30 http://www.theguardian.com/society/2014/apr/01/nhs-chief-simon-stevens-private-innovation?CMP=twt_gu.

31 http://www.theguardian.com/politics/2014/sep/06/lynton-crosby-lobbied-for-tobacco-giant-philip-morris.

32 http://www.newstatesman.com/politics/2014/06/we-need-talk-about-nhs-cameron-must-break-crosby-imposed-silence.

33 http://www.theguardian.com/technology/2006/sep/28/news.business.

34 http://www.theregister.co.uk/2006/09/29/accenture_nhs_penalty/.

35 http://www.telegraph.co.uk/news/uknews/1473927/Bill-for-hi-tech-NHS-soars-to-20-billion.html.

36 http://www.nao.org.uk/report/department-of-health-the-national-programme-for-it-in-the-nhs/.

37 http://www.legislation.gov.uk/ukpga/2012/7/part/9/enacted.

38 http://www.dailymail.co.uk/news/article-2315003/U-turn-NHS-database-opt-Victory-privacy-campaign-Hunt-backs-down.html.

39 http://www.england.nhs.uk/2013/10/16/care-data/.

40 http://en.wikipedia.org/wiki/List_of_UK_government_data_losses.

41 http://www.theguardian.com/society/2014/jan/19/nhs-patient-data-available-companies-buy.

42 ttp://systems.hscic.gov.uk/scr.

43 http://www.newstatesman.com/politics/2014/06/why-tories-have-stopped-talking-about-nhs; http://www.leftfutures.org/2014/09/leaks-show-us-multinationals-now-directing-doctors-commissioning-groups/.

44 http://www.theguardian.com/society/2014/aug/30/nhs-bosses-summits-contracts-unitedhealth-insurer.

45 Leys, Colin & Player, Stewart, 2011. p. 6.

46 http://www.telegraph.co.uk/news/politics/9722661/David-Cameron-ordered-to-stop-saying-NHS-spending-is-up.html.

47 http://skwalker1964.wordpress.com/2013/06/12/cameron-repeats-his-nhs-12-7bn-lie-in-pmqs-twice-help-shut-him-down/.

48 http://www.greenbenchesuk.com/2013/11/jeremy-hunts-latest-lie-is-insult-to.htm; http://www.walesonline.co.uk/news/wales-news/your-party-told-tissue-lies-7973329.

49 Leys, Colin & Player, Stewart, 2011. p. 6.
50 Paton, Calum, 2014. *At what cost? Paying the price for the market in the English NHS*, London: Centre for Health and the Public Interest http://chpi.org.uk/wp-content/uploads/2014/02/At-what-cost-paying-the-price-for-the-market-in-the-English-NHS-by-Calum-Paton.pdf.

Chapter 12

1   'NHS reforms our worst mistake, Tories admit.' *The Times*, 1 and 13 October 2014, http://www.thetimes.co.uk/tto/news/politics/article4234883.ece
2   Appleby J. 2013. 'Spending on health and social care over the next 50 years, Why think long term?' King's Fund, http://www.kingsfund.org.uk/sites/files/kf/field/field_publication_file/Spending per cent20on per cent20health per cent20... per cent2050 per cent20years per cent20low per cent20res per cent20for per cent20web.pdf.
3   Helm T, Campbell D. 2014. 'GP numbers tumble in England as recruitment crisis bites', *The Observer*, 14 June, http://www.theguardian.com/society/2014/jun/14/gp-numbers-fall-recruitment-crisis-bites; Cooper C. 2014. 'District nurses could be a thing of the past in 10 years without urgent action, warns Royal College of Nurses', *The Independent*, June 17, http://www.independent.co.uk/life-style/health-and-families/health-news/district-nurses-could-be-a-thing-of-the-past-in-10-years-without-urgent-action-warns-royal-college-of-nurses-9541526.html.
4   Ham C. 2014. 'The NHS is more fragmented than ever: Are ministers prepared to provide the means required to deliver integrated care?' *The Independent*, 14 January 2014, http://www.independent.co.uk/voices/comment/the-nhs-is-more-fragmented-than-ever-9057015.html.
5   Lintern S. 2014. 'Exclusive: Staff shortage fuels recruitment of nearly 6,000 overseas nurses', *HSJ*, 17 December, http://www.hsj.co.uk/news/exclusive-staff-shortage-fuels-recruitment-of-nearly-6000-overseas-nurses/5077720.article?blocktitle=Nursing-news&contentID=1745#.VJcJjDpACg.
6   McNicoll A. 2014. 'Mentally unwell children sent hundreds of miles for care amid bed shortage' *Community Care*, February 20, 2014, http://www.communitycare.co.uk/2014/02/20/mentally-ill-children-sent-hundreds-miles-care-due-bed-shortage/.
7   Lister J. 2014a. *London's NHS at the Crossroads, Executive summary*, Unite the Union, March, http://www.peoplesinquiry.org.uk/pdf/NHSattheCrossroadsExecsummary.pdf.

8   Syal R. 2014. 'Half of councils at risk of financial failure within five years, say auditors', *The Guardian*, 19 November, http://www.theguardian.com/society/2014/nov/19/councils-risk-financial-failure-auditors.

9   Williams D. 2014. 'Exclusive: Better care fund investment returns 'wildly unrealistic', analysis finds', *HSJ* 18 December, http://www.hsj.co.uk/news/finance/exclusive-better-care-fund-investment-returns-wildly-unrealistic-analysis-finds/5077756.article#.VJcOLDpAGg.

10   Available http://www.healthemergency.org.uk/pdf/McKinsey%20affordability%20document%20for%20NHS%20London%202009.pdf

11   Partnerships Bulletin. 2014. 'Miliband offers PFI defence', 9 December, http://www.partnershipsbulletin.com/news/view/85000.

12   Monbiot G. 2010. *The UK's Odious Debts*, November 22, http://www.monbiot.com/2010/11/22/the-uks-odious-debts/.

13   http://www.ft.com/cms/s/0/cc4f10b2-4951-11e4-8d68-00144feab7de.html#axzz3MYkDs2Nz.

14   http://www.peoplesvotefornhs.org.uk/pledges.

15   Lister J. 2014b. *Preliminary Briefing to People's Inquiry Panel*, December 2014 http://www.peoplesinquiry.org/pdf/Sections%20from%20initial%20Panel%20Briefing.pdf .

16   http://www.england.nhs.uk/wp-content/uploads/2014/10/5yfv-web.pdf.

17   http://www.telegraph.co.uk/news/nhs/11182590/The-health-revolution-is-under-way-but-no-fanfare-please.html.

18   https://www.opendemocracy.net/ournhs/shibley-rahman/nhs-five-year-forward-view-wishlist-for-privatisers.

19   http://www.independent.co.uk/life-style/health-and-families/health-news/alarm-at-surprise-fall-in-life-expectancy-amid-fears-that-cuts-and-pressure-on-nhs-may-be-to-blame-for-earlier-deaths-9973848.html.

20   Lister J. 2014c, 'A blow against privatisation', *Morning Star*, October 21, http://www.morningstaronline.co.uk/a-627a-A-blow-against-privatisation#.VJcvvDpAGg.

21   http://www.bbc.co.uk/news/uk-england-29094093.

22   Iacobucci G. 2014. 'A third of NHS contracts awarded since health act have hone to private sector', *BMJ*, 10 December, doi: http://dx.doi.org/10.1136/bmj.g7606.

23   Stoye G. 2013. 'Public payment and private provision: the changing landscape of healthcare in the 2000s', Institute for Fiscal Studies, May 2013.

24   http://www.healthinvestor.co.uk/ShowArticle.aspx?ID=3501&AspxAutoDetectCookieSupport=1.

25   http://www.westbriton.co.uk/Privatisation-fears-75million-NHS-services/story-21299045-detail/story.html.

26 https://www.facebook.com/cancernotforprofit.

27 e.g. www.nhsbill2015.org/.

28 Campbell D. 2014. 'Half of voters happy to pay more tax to fund NHS – poll', *The Guardian*, Friday 15 August, available http://www.theguardian.com/society/2014/aug/15/voters-tax-fund-nhs-poll.

29 Milne S. 2012. 'A roll call of corporate rogues who are milking the country', *The Guardian*, 30 October, available http://www.theguardian.com/commentisfree/2012/oct/30/roll-call-corporate-rogues-tax.

30 http://policy.greenparty.org.uk/he.html.

31 http://nhap.org/our-policies-1/ .

32 http://www.nhsbill2015.org/category/news/page/3/.

33 http://www.theguardian.com/society/2015/jan/09/circle-hospital-private-firms-nhs-report-poor-care-hinchingbrooke.

34 Ibid.

35 http://www.dailymail.co.uk/news/article-2632191/Private-firm-turned-failing-NHS-hospital-award-winner-From-basket-case-best-country-patient-care.html.

36 http://www.dailymail.co.uk/news/article-2905936/There-s-no-reason-pull-plug-miracle-hospital-say-patients-suspicion-mounts-privately-run-hospital-stitched-up.html.

37 https://www.opendemocracy.net/ournhs/caroline-molloy/hinchingbrooke-why-did-england per cent27s-privatised-hospital-deal-really-collapse.

38 http://news.rapgenius.com/Noam-chomsky-the-state-corporate-complex-a-threat-to-freedom-and-survival-annotated#

Appendix I

1 David Cameron speech 'Rebuilding Trust in Politics', 8 February 2010.

2 United Health Group website, accessed January 2015 http://www.unitedhealthgroup.com/Businesses/Optum.aspx.

3 United Health Group website, accessed January 2015 http://www.unitedhealthgroup.com/Home/About/Default.aspx.

4 Gallager P. 'Is Simon Stevens really the right person to run the NHS?', *Independent,* 24 October 2013: http://www.independent.co.uk/news/uk/politics/is-simon-stevens-really-the-right-person-to-run-the-nhs-8902251.html; Miller V and Feeley J. 'UnitedHealth to Pay $500 Million Over Hepatitis Doctor', *Bloomberg,* 10 April 2013: http://www.bloomberg.com/news/2013-04-09/unitedhealth-to-pay-500-million-over-hepatitis-doctor.html; Inman P. 'UnitedHealth: Big profits but some questions', *Guardian,* 16 July 2010: http://www.theguardian.com/

politics/2010/jul/16/unitedhealth-profits-questions.

5   UnitedHealth Group profile, OpenSecrets.org; https://www.opensecrets.org/orgs/summary.php?cycle=2014&id=D000000348.

6   Paduano M. 'Private companies on Staffordshire cancer contract shortlist', BBC website, 6 November 2014: http://www.bbc.co.uk/news/uk-england-stoke-staffordshire-29929934.

7   Email from Christopher Exeter, United Health lobbyist, to Bob Ricketts, NHS England, 25 April 2014: document received under FOI law from NHS England.

8   Ibid.

9   Doward J. 'Calls for greater disclosure on NHS chiefs' meetings with private US health insurer', *Observer*, 30 August 2014: http://www.theguardian.com/society/2014/aug/30/nhs-bosses-summits-contracts-unitedhealth-insurer.

10   Ibid.

11   Foot T. 'Over here... US team drafted onto board of firm running GP surgeries', *Camden New Journal*, 3 July 2008: http://www.thecnj.com/camden/2008/070308/news070308_03.html.

12   Hanover Communications entries on the Association of Professional Political Consultants' voluntary register of lobbyists: http://www.appc.org.uk/members/.

13   NHS England spending data 2013-14: http://www.england.nhs.uk/contact-us/pub-scheme/spend/#payments.

14   Harrison A. 'The Simon Stevens I worked with at the Department of Health', Hanover Communications blog, 24 October 2013: http://www.hanovercomms.com/2013/10/the-simon-stevens-i-worked-with-at-the-department-of-health/#sthash.DfUUMe3v.dpuf.

15   Ramesh R. 'Private healthcare group lobbied competition body for NHS inquiry', *Guardian*, 29 July 2011: http://www.theguardian.com/society/2011/jul/29/prk.

16   NHS Partners Network, 'Director's update on the NHS Reforms', 20 May 2011, released by the NHS Partners Network.

17   Ibid.

18   'Transparency', Reform website, accessed January 2015: http://www.reform.co.uk/about/transparency/.

19   Cave T and Rowell A. *A Quiet Word*, Vintage, 2014, pp. 132-4.

20   'About Us' and 'Our supporters', Cambridge Health Network website, accessed January 2015: http://cambridgehealthnetwork.com/about-us/; 'http://cambridgehealthnetwork.com/about-us/supporters/; Cambridge Health Network, Judge Business School website, accessed January 2015: http://www.health.jbs.cam.ac.uk/corporate/outreach.html.

21 'Events', Cambridge Health Network website, accessed January 2015: http://cambridgehealthnetwork.com/events/previous-events/page/3/

22 Penny Dash is also a former Trustee and Vice Chair of the King's Fund, former Head of Strategy for the NHS, and headed the McKinsey team working with then Labour minister Lord Darzi on his Next Stage Review. http://www.nuffieldtrust.org.uk/summit/2011/speakers/dr-penny-dash.

22 'Our Team', Cambridge Health Network website, accessed January 2015: http://cambridgehealthnetwork.com/about-us/our-team/.

23 Player S, and Leys C. 'Dismantling the NHS', *Red Pepper*, October 2010: http://www.redpepper.org.uk/dismantling-the-nhs/.

24 'Spending over £25,000', April 2013 to April 2014; data releases by Department of Health, NHS England; and Monitor.

25 Rose D. 'The firm that hijacked the NHS', *Mail on Sunday*, 12 February 2012.

26 Email from 'MM' at McKinsey to David Bennet and Adrian Masters of Monitor, 31 May 2010, received under FOI law from Monitor.

27 Ramesh R. 'German company involved in talks to take over NHS hospitals', *Guardian*, 4 September 2011, based on documents released under FOI law to Tamasin Cave by the Department of Health: http://www.theguardian.com/society/2011/sep/04/german-company-takeover-nhs-hospitals.

28 NHS England spending data 2013-14: http://www.england.nhs.uk/contact-us/pub-scheme/spend/#payments.

29 Ibid.

30 Doward J. 'Calls for greater disclosure on NHS chiefs' meetings with private US health insurer', *Observer*, 30 August 2014: http://www.theguardian.com/society/2014/aug/30/nhs-bosses-summits-contracts-unitedhealth-insurer.

31 Apax Global Healthcare Services Conference, 'Opportunities Post Global Healthcare Reforms', October 2010: http://powerbase.info/images/f/fe/Apax_Healthcare_conference_2010.pdf.

32 Reed K. 'Alan Milburn takes PwC health role', *Accountancy Age*, 23 May 2013 http://www.accountancyage.com/aa/news/2270407/alan-milburn-takes-pwc-health-role.

33 John S. *The Persuaders: When Lobbyists Matter*, Palgrave Macmillan, 2002, p. 52.

34 Novatis' entries on the voluntary registers of lobbyists operated by the Association of Professional Political Consultants and the Public Relations Consultants Association: http://www.appc.org.uk/members/; http://www.prca.org.uk/paregister.

35 Memorandum from The Association of the British Pharmaceutical

Industry to the Public Administration Select Committee, May 2008:
http://www.parliament.the-stationery-office.com/pa/cm200809/cmselect/
cmpubadm/36/36we15.htm.

Appendix 2

1   http://www.nhsforsale.info/uploads/images/contract%20alert%20re-
    port%20Apr-Apr%20final%20(1).pdf.
2   http://www.nhscampaign.org/about/briefings-and-documents/nhs-
    unlimited.html.
3   http://www.telegraph.co.uk/journalists/laura-donnelly/10730105/NHS-
    spending-doubles-on-private-ambulances-used-for-999-calls.html.
4   http://www.bbc.co.uk/news/uk-england-cornwall-25362545.
5   http://www.nhsforsale.info/private-providers/private-provider-profiles-2/
    care-uk.html.
6   http://ted.europa.eu/udl?uri=TED:NOTICE:234407-
    2014:TEXT:EN:HTML&tabId=1.
7   http://www.hscic.gov.uk.
8   http://www.hscic.gov.uk.
9   http://www.theguardian.com/society/2012/nov/19/nhs-patients-treated-
    private-firms.
10 http://ted.europa.eu/udl?uri=TED:NOTICE:199182-
    2014:TEXT:EN:HTML&src=0.
11 http://ted.europa.eu/udl?uri=TED:NOTICE:241100-
    2014:TEXT:EN:HTML&src=0.
12 http://www.theguardian.com/uk-news/2014/jul/02/cancer-care-nhs-out-
    sourcing-ccgs-unison-virgin.
13 http://www.ft.com/cms/s/0/657b30e6-357a-11e3-952b-00144feab7de.
    html#axzz3FXyKIDZ8.
14 http://www.ft.com/cms/s/0/bcf1269c-9e1a-11e3-95fe-00144feab7de.
    html#axzz3FXyKIDZ8.
15 http://ted.europa.eu/udl?uri=TED:NOTICE:340941-
    2013:TEXT:EN:HTML&src=0.
16 http://www.theguardian.com/business/2013/jul/18/bain-capital-plasma-
    resources-uk.
17 See for example: https://www.opendemocracy.net/ourkingdom/clare-
    sambrook/pfi-transferring-billions-from-uk-taxpayers-to-private-finan-
    ciers; Mark Hellowell and Allyson M. Pollock, 'The Private Financing of
    NHS Hospitals: Politics, Policy And Practice', www.sps.ed.ac.uk/__data/
    assets/pdf_file/0020/64352/econ_affairs.pdf; 'NHS faces £65bn bill for
    PFI hospitals', http://www.theguardian.com/politics/2010/aug/13/nhs-pfi-

65-billion-bill-repayments; http://www.bbc.co.uk/news/health-10882522.

18 https://www.opendemocracy.net/ournhs/david-lock/nhs-competition-regulations-response-to-governments-attacks.

19 http://www.nhsforsale.info/uploads/images/contract%20alert%20report%20Apr-Apr%20final%20(1).pdf.

20 http://www.gponline.com/services-open-any-qualified-provider-revealed-dh/article/1149786.

21 http://www.theguardian.com/society/2014/oct/10/advances-nhs-care-reverse.

22 http://www.theguardian.com/society/2014/dec/09/nhs-management-consultants-bill-doubles-640m.

23 *The Mirror:* 31 March 2014, http://www.mirror.co.uk/news/uk-news/top-cancer-doctors-damning-letter-3320345.

24 BMJ: 8 September 2014.

25 'Measuring up? The health of NHS cancer services', Cancer Research UK, http://www.cancerresearchuk.org/sites/default/files/measuring_up_health_of_nhs_cancer_services_sept2014.pdf.

26 22 September 2014, *The Guardian,* http://www.theguardian.com/society/patrick-butler-cuts-blog/2014/sep/22/outsourcing-same-job-same-hours-less-pay.

27 http://www.theguardian.com/society/disability.

28 http://www.theguardian.com/society/2014/nov/16/nhs-trusts-chasing-private-patients.

29 http://www.theguardian.com/society/2015/jan/07/patients-hospital-elderly-bedblockers-care-, http://www.bbc.co.uk/news/health-30742817.

30 http://www.independent.co.uk/life-style/health-and-families/health-news/thousands-of-patients-at-risk-from-nhs-outsourcing-9799937.html.

31 http://www.hsj.co.uk/news/commissioning/ccgs-open-services-to-competition-out-of-fear-of-rules/5069521.article#.VM4doY1ybxk

32 http://www.theguardian.com/society/2014/apr/04/gp-local-nhs-forced-health-services-tender.

33 *Pharma Times,* 10 September 2014, http://www.pharmatimes.com/article/14-09-10/vast_majority_of_nhs_staff_say_reform_had_negative_impact.aspx.

34 http://www.theguardian.com/society/2014/oct/23/nhs-paid-service-public-fears.

35 http://www.pulsetoday.co.uk/commissioning/85-of-gps-believe-nhs-will-be-privatised-within-ten-years/20007870.article#VK6GsdKsWIB.

36 http://www.pulsetoday.co.uk/home/finance-and-practice-life-news/practice-survey-reveals-just-one-fifth-of-gps-expect-their-practice-to-survive/20007592.article#.VM4iC41ybxk.

37 http://www.hsj.co.uk/news/junior-doctors-raise-patient-care-con-
    cerns/5073656.article#.VK53IdKsWlA.
38 http://www.dailymail.co.uk/wires/pa/article-2717713/Junior-doctors-
    start-.
39 http://www.hsj.co.uk/news/keep-politics-out-of-nhs-says-poll/5072226.
    article#.VK5329KsWlA.

Index

About the Authors

Tamasin Cave is a writer and campaigner. She is director of Spinwatch, which investigates corporate PR and lobbying, http://www.spinwatch.org/, and the co-author of *A Quiet Word: Lobbying, Crony Capitalism, and Broken Politics in Britain*, Vintage, 2014.

Dr Jacky Davis is a consultant radiologist in north London. She co-edited *NHS SOS*, is a founder member of Keep our NHS Public and is a member of the BMA UK council.

Paul Evans is a director of the NHS Support Federation, a pressure group founded to protect the principles of the NHS. He has worked on campaigns and research across the voluntary sector and in Parliament.

Dr John Lister, Director of London Health Emergency since 1984, is a founder member of Keep Our NHS Public, a public speaker, journalist, and author of books on the NHS, global health and health journalism.

Prof. Martin McKee CBE is Professor of European Public Health at the London School of Hygiene and Tropical Medicine. In 2014 he was named as one of the three most highly cited researchers on global health systems research.

Harry Smith is a survivor of the Great Depression, a Second World War RAF veteran and, at 91, an activist for the poor and for the preservation of social democracy. He has authored numerous books about Britain during the Great Depression, the Second World War and post-war austerity. He lives outside Toronto, Canada and in Yorkshire.

Dr David Wrigley is a GP in Carnforth, Lancashire. He speaks for Keep Our NHS Public and is a member of the BMA UK Council and BMA General Practitioners Committee.